Hortense Cotrim

Efficacy of Acupuncture in Carpal Canal Syndrome

Hortense Cotrim

Efficacy of Acupuncture in Carpal Canal Syndrome

Research Protocol

ScienciaScripts

Imprint
Any brand names and product names mentioned in this book are subject to trademark, brand or patent protection and are trademarks or registered trademarks of their respective holders. The use of brand names, product names, common names, trade names, product descriptions etc. even without a particular marking in this work is in no way to be construed to mean that such names may be regarded as unrestricted in respect of trademark and brand protection legislation and could thus be used by anyone.

Cover image: www.ingimage.com

This book is a translation from the original published under ISBN 978-613-9-65613-4.

Publisher:
Sciencia Scripts
is a trademark of
Dodo Books Indian Ocean Ltd. and OmniScriptum S.R.L publishing group

120 High Road, East Finchley, London, N2 9ED, United Kingdom
Str. Armeneasca 28/1, office 1, Chisinau MD-2012, Republic of Moldova, Europe
Printed at: see last page
ISBN: 978-620-7-79226-9

CONTENTS

ACKNOWLEDGMENTS...2
SUMMARY...3
INTRODUCTION...4
1. STATE OF THE ART 6
2. TRADITIONAL CHINESE MEDICINE 14
3. METHODOLOGY 23
4. Discussion and Conclusions 50
5. BIBLIOGRAPHICAL REFERENCES 55
6. ANNEXES 59

The greatest reward for

man's work is not what he gets out of it,

but what he becomes out of it.

John Ruskin

ACKNOWLEDGMENTS

I believe that any dissertation is the product of the collective effort of a large group of people, whose guidance, commitment and dedication contribute greatly to its completion. To all of them I express my deepest gratitude:

To Professor **Jorge Machado**, co-supervisor of this study, for the support, encouragement and trust he has always shown me.

To Master **Maria Joao Santos**, the supervisor of this study, whose criticisms and suggestions gave quality to this work. Her dedication, insight and willingness to teach have borne fruit.

To **my colleagues on** this journey, for their availability and encouragement at different times and unconditionally.

To the **friends and clients** who believed in my knowledge and allowed me to evolve and learn the basics of acupuncture, which led me to carry out this study. I would also like to thank them for so readily agreeing to answer the questionnaires, using up some of their time, which is already so scarce.

To the memory of my father, **Américo,** and my mother, **Delfina**, for their wise lessons in hope; for the love and courage they always passed on to me, giving me the confidence to set off in search of my dreams.

To my sons, **Bruno**, **Carlos** and **Nuno,** who continue to give me the strongest reason to celebrate family. You are the deepest lesson in ethics, dignity and love...

To my husband, **Carlos**, for his love, unconditional support and trust. For everything and everything else, here is my deepest affection.

SUMMARY

Carpal tunnel syndrome is a peripheral neuropathy resulting from compression of the median nerve, which passes through a narrow tunnel located in the wrist region, known as the carpal tunnel.

Compression is caused by enlargement or thickening of the structures that pass through the tunnel. It is often related to manual labor, with prolonged repetition of movements, which leads to repetitive strain injury. However, it is also associated with other hormonal changes, such as the menopause and pregnancy, which explains its higher incidence in women aged between 35 and 60. Other possible causes are obesity, diabetes, thyroid disease and rheumatoid arthritis, among others.

The most common symptoms are pain, numbness, tingling and reduced manual dexterity, which occur more frequently at night.

Acupuncture aims to establish the circulation of energy (Qi) and blood in the body, thus leading to harmony between energy and matter, the constituents of the human body. The aim of this study was to find out whether this balance provided by acupuncture helps to reduce the symptoms of Carpal Canal Syndrome.

The clinical cases presented point in this direction, since all the patients showed a significant reduction in symptoms, as well as a marked improvement in manual dexterity and grip strength, which allowed them to carry out their activities of daily living satisfactorily.

It should be noted, however, that there is still little rigorous scientific evidence on the effect of acupuncture in controlling the symptoms of this pathology. Despite this fact, several studies show that acupuncture is successful in treating various pathologies and is especially effective in controlling pain.

We selected the Boston Self-Assessment Questionnaire as the measuring instrument. A dynamometer was used to assess grip strength.

Key words: Carpal Canal Syndrome, Traditional Chinese Medicine, Acupuncture.

The qi can't travel without a path, just as water flows or the moon orbits without resting. Thus, the Yin vessels nourish the zang and the yang vessels nourish thefu.

(Deadman et al, 2012)

INTRODUCTION

Carpal canal syndrome (CCS) is a compression neuropathy of the median nerve at the wrist and the most common of the entrapment neuropathies (Nobuta et al, 2008). It is included in the group of musculoskeletal diseases, which are the main cause of chronic pain, absenteeism from work and temporary or permanent disability (Bugajska et al, 2007).

It is a painful condition that occurs predominantly in adults between the ages of 40 and 60, is 5 times more common in women than in men and is very rare in children (Banner & Hudson, 2001).

It is characterized by symptomatic compression of the median nerve, whose main symptoms include an unpleasant sensation of tingling, pain and/or numbness in the distal part of the upper extremities, corresponding to the areas where the median nerve is distributed, namely the thumb, index, middle and radial part of the ring finger, as well as reduced strength and function of the affected hand, (Yunoki et al, 2017).

Given the disability that this pathology imposes on a population that is mostly active, it is very important to find therapeutic measures that respond to the need to reduce the associated symptoms. Conventional therapy doesn't provide definitive and lasting answers, whether surgical or conservative, so a multidisciplinary approach is imperative in order to improve the quality of life of individuals with this syndrome. This is where acupuncture comes in, as a way of helping to alleviate the symptoms of CCS and improve the activities of daily living of those affected.

In this sense, Khosrawi and colleagues (2012) carried out a randomized controlled study to evaluate the effectiveness of acupuncture in improving the symptoms associated with carpal tunnel syndrome, concluding that acupuncture can reduce the symptoms associated with the condition overall, and can be included in patients' recovery programs.

Although there is some controversy in the literature regarding the effectiveness of acupuncture in controlling pain, some studies have already shown positive results, such as the randomized study carried out by Berman and colleagues (2004), on patients with osteoarthritis of the knee, in which it was found that patients who received 8 weeks of acupuncture experienced significant improvements in the movement of the joint and a significant reduction in pain, when compared to patients who received sham acupuncture.

Chung and colleagues (2016) also found, in their study of patients with primary CCS, with mild to moderate but chronic symptoms and no indication for surgery, that electroacupuncture produced small improvements in symptoms, as well as in functional capacity, manual dexterity and *grip strength,* when combined with the use of an immobilizing splint at night.

4

In this context, a study based on clinical cases was carried out with the aim of evaluating the effect of acupuncture on the painful and functional symptoms associated with carpal tunnel syndrome. The results obtained in the treatment of 4 patients with carpal tunnel syndrome were presented, 2 with and 2 without surgical indication. The patients without a surgical indication had their wrists immobilized with a splint at night and for long periods during the day. This study was carried out in a clinical setting at Clinica Carlos Cotrim II - Cuidados de Saù, Lda, where the patients voluntarily agreed to take part in the study.

1. STATE OF THE ART

1.1 Carpal Cane Syndrome

The carpal canal is the anatomical region where the flexor tendons of the fingers and the median nerve are located. The roof of the canal is formed by the flexor retinaculum or transverse carpal ligament. The retinaculum is a fibrous band 2.5 to 3.5 mm thick and 3 to 4 cm wide, immediately above the median nerve, at the level of the wrist (Meirelles et al.; 2006).

Carpal canal syndrome is one of the most common compressive neuropathies of the upper extremities, caused by compression of the median nerve, which travels through the carpal canal, causing pain, tingling sensations and numbness throughout the area that it supplies, including the palmar area of the thumb, index and middle fingers and the radial part of the ring finger (Wipperman & Goerl; 2016).

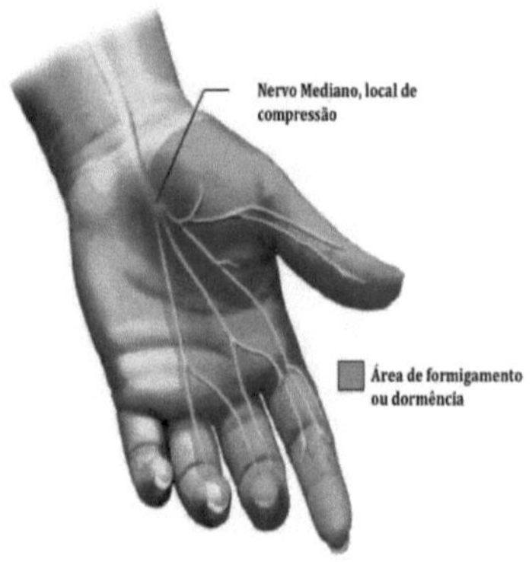

FIGURA 1: The carpal tunnel syndrome. Site of compression of the median nerve.

Source: http://www.spclinic.pt/tratamento-sindrome-canal-carpico/

From a pathophysiological point of view, compressive syndromes combine the phenomena of compression and tension. Anatomically, there are two sites of compression of the median nerve: one at the level of the proximal limit of the carpal tunnel, caused by wrist flexion due to changes in the thickness and stiffness of the forearm fascia and the proximal portion of the flexor retinaculum; and the second at the level of the narrowest portion, near the hamate hook, (Chammas et al, 2014).

As a way of better characterizing this pathology from a pathophysiological point of view, Meirelles et al. (2006) point out that it is characterized by compression of the median nerve in the area where it crosses the carpal region. Compression can occur due to a decrease in the interior of the canal or an increase in the volume of the structures contained within it. Anatomical studies show that the narrowest region of the tunnel is distal to the level of the hamate and that during wrist flexion the nerve is compressed by the proximal margin of the flexor retinaculum.

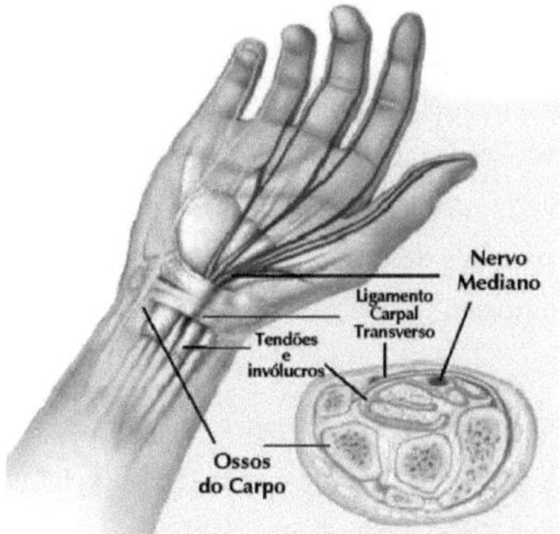

FIGURA 2:   Anatomy of the carpal tunnel

Source: http://www.ricardokaempf.com.br/

Carpal tunnel syndrome is divided into three stages, depending on the severity of the symptoms. Yunoki et al. (2017) state that based on clinical symptoms, stage 1 includes patients who wake up with a feeling of numbness or swelling of the hand, but without visible edema. These patients often report that shaking or tapping the hand eliminates the pain, although a certain stiffness remains during the morning. The same authors state that the second stage involves the continuation of these symptoms during the day and the third stage occurs when there is already hypotrophy or atrophy of the tenar muscle. In this stage, users also report a decrease in hand strength, which makes it difficult to carry out daily tasks.

For their part, Chammas and colleagues (2014) also presented a clinical-anatomical classification of the pathology, based on the symptoms presented. These authors point out that compression and traction of the nerve can sequentially create problems related to intraneural blood microcirculation, damage to the myelin sheath and axonal level and changes in the supporting connective tissue. Thus, based on these alterations, the authors consider that the initial stage is characterized by intermittent symptoms that only occur at night; the intermediate stage, in which the symptoms are nocturnal and diurnal. Microcirculation abnormalities are constantly present, with epineural and intrafascicular interstitial edema, which causes an increase in endoneural fluid pressure; finally the advanced stage, in which symptoms are constantly present, especially signs of sensory or motor deficit, reflected in the interruption of a greater or lesser number of axons. Once the nerve has been released, recovery depends on the regeneration of the nerve, which takes several months and may be incomplete. The significance of recovery will depend on the patient's potential for axonal regeneration, particularly in relation to age, the existence of polyneuropathy and the severity of the compression.

As far as symptoms are concerned, Yunoki and colleagues (2017) state that the main symptoms are a reduction in the strength and function of the affected hand. Compression can occur due to a decrease in the interior of the canal or an increase in the volume of the structures contained within it (Meirelles et al.; 2006). Symptoms tend to worsen during the night and an important aspect of the diagnosis is the fact that the patient wakes up during the night as a result of the manifestation and/or worsening of symptoms. Still on the subject of diagnosis, Yunoki and colleagues (2017) state that the diagnosis is often made on the basis of the patient's description, which states that, in addition to the aspects described above, it is customary to relieve the pain by shaking the wrist, or by giving the sore area a little tap.

This syndrome is included in musculoskeletal diseases, which are the main cause of chronic pain and absenteeism from work, affecting the quality of life of individuals, mainly due to the associated temporary or permanent incapacity to carry out activities (Bugajska et al; 2007). Leigh and colleagues (2011) also state that since this is a work-related pathology, it has a marked economic impact, often with workers demanding monetary compensation. There are numerous activities that are related to the onset of CCS, particularly those that require repetitive movements, the use of force and awkward hand positions (Bugajska et al, 2007).

1.1.1. Incidence and Prevalence

The figures found in terms of incidence and prevalence of this pathology demonstrate its importance to the medical community.

Chammas and colleagues (2014) report that the estimated prevalence of CCS in the general population varies between 4% and 5% and particularly affects individuals aged between 40 and 60. The same authors point out that, in 2008, 127,269 individuals aged 20 or over underwent surgical intervention to treat CCS in metropolitan France, giving an incidence of 2.7/1000 (Women: 3.6/1000; Men: 1.7/1000). They also point out that there are two peaks of frequency, the first and highest being between the ages of 49 and 59, in which the vast majority (75%) are women; and the second peak is between the ages of 75 and 84, in which women account for 64%. Yunoki et al. (2017) also report that 1 to 4% of the general population suffers from this condition, with 1 to 2 individuals out of every 5 suffering from symptoms of pain, tingling and numbness in the upper extremities being diagnosed with carpal tunnel syndrome. The annual incidence of this condition is 276/100,000 inhabitants. The same authors point out that it is more common in women, with a two-thirds to one-third ratio between women and men. Mondelli and colleagues (2002) state that the development of this pathology is also related to age. Although it is seen in all age groups, it has a higher incidence in the 40-60 age group. The same authors point out that only 10% occur before the age of 30. In the same vein, Bugajska et al. (2007) add that the incidence also increases with the number of years worked. It should be noted that the fact that the pathology is more common in the elderly means that there is a more marked decrease in the mobility and independence of the elderly in carrying out activities of daily living.

In order to emphasize the importance of this pathology, Prime and colleagues (2010) point out that the prevalence of CFS in the general population is 2.7%. In the UK, it is 7-16%, which corresponds to an average of 26 days off work per year; these authors also present estimates from the USA for 1995, where between 400,000 and 500,000 users underwent carpal tunnel decompression surgery, which corresponds to an economic cost of 2 billion dollars.

As a way of emphasizing the importance of this pathology, Ashworth (2009) states that it has an incidence of 105 cases per 100,000 inhabitants per year. For males, the incidence is 52 cases per 100,000 inhabitants and for females it is 149 cases per 100,000 inhabitants per year. With regard to age, the same author states that the incidence increases with age in males, while in females the incidence is higher between the ages of 45 and 54.

1.1.2. Triggering Factors

Carpal canal syndrome is the most common compressive syndrome and its most common cause is idiopathic. With regard to idiopathic syndromes, Chammas and colleagues (2014) point out that they occur more frequently in women (65-80%), between the ages of 40 and 60, and are bilateral in 50 to 60% of cases. Although spontaneous regression is possible, worsening symptoms are the rule. Diagnosis is primarily clinical, based on symptoms and clinical observation maneuvers designed to confirm the diagnosis. An electroneuromyographic examination may be recommended preoperatively or in the case of occupational disease (Chammas et al, 2014).

Aroori and Spense (2008) consider that there are two varieties of this syndrome, acute and chronic, pointing out that the acute form is relatively uncommon and is due to a rapid and sustained increase in pressure in the carpal tunnel. This cause is generally associated with a fracture of the radius, although it can also be associated with burns, coagulopathy, local infection or the injection of substances. Chronic pain is much more common, with symptoms persisting for months or years. However, the aforementioned authors point out that only in 50% of cases are the causes identified. These can be local, regional or systemic.

Thus, and based on the opinion of Aroori and Spense (2008), we can point to the following as local causes:

- Inflammatory: tenosynovitis, histoplasma infection, synovial hypertrophy;

- Trauma: Colles' fracture, dislocation of one of the carpal bones

- Tumors: hemangioma, cysts, ganglia, lipomas, neuromas, etc.

- Anatomical changes: thickening of the transverse carpal ligament, bone anomalies, muscle anomalies, persistent median artery, etc.

As regional causes, the same authors highlight:

- Osteoarthritis;

- Rheumatoid arthritis;

- Amyloidosis;

- Drop.

Systemic causes include

- Diabetes;

- Obesity;

- Hypothyroidism;

- Pregnancy;

- Menopause;

- Systemic lupus erythematosus;

- Scleroderma;

- Dermatomyositis;

- Renal failure;

- Hemodialysis for prolonged periods;

- Acromegaly;

- Multiple myeloma;

- Sarcoidosis;

- Leukemia;

- Alcoholism;

- Hemophilia (Aroori & Spense, 2008).

In order to better understand this pathology, we can say that the causes of CCS can be general or local. In the case of generalized causes, the neuropathy derives from the narrowing of the carpal canal, which causes an increase in tissue pressure due to the development of connective tissue or the formation of crystal deposits and its origin is related to hormonal changes (acromegaly or hypothyroidism), pregnancy and the menopause, metabolic diseases (diabetes, amyloidosis, obesity, mucopolysaccharidosis and pseudogout), blood vessel diseases (hypertension, Raynaud's syndrome and thrombosis of the median artery) and others, such as allergic reactions (Bugajska et al, 2007). The same authors point out that local causes include deformation of the bony elements of the carpal canal due to trauma, deep burn scars, degenerative and inflammatory changes in the tendon sheaths, malformation of the muscles, bones and vessels of the wrist joint, tumors and para-tumors, as well as mycotic lesions.

For their part, Yunoki and colleagues (2017) point out that CCS remains an idiopathic disease, although some risk factors can be identified, which can be divided into 3 categories: anatomical, mechanical and physiological. Thus, anatomical factors are related to the fact that the carpal canal is narrower in some people than in others, which is why this pathology is more common in women. Other abnormalities, such as the appearance of ganglia, cysts and tumors, which will cause an increase in the pressure of the interstitial fluids. Trauma can also cause restriction of the volume of the canal due to the presence of hemorrhage, distortion of anatomical structures or the formation of scars.

These authors point out that the main mechanical factors are those related to professional activities, such as repetitive movements that require continuous effort, or activities that involve constant vibration of the hand and wrist. For this reason, the dominant hand is generally the most affected, although it is common for symptoms to be present in both hands, particularly if the cause of the pathology is related to anatomical factors. The non-dominant hand can also be affected in patients whose dominant hand is incapacitated, as in the case of strokes or tremors due to Parkinson's disease. Finally, there are the physiological factors, which are associated with medical conditions such as obesity, drug intoxication, alcoholism, diabetes, hypothyroidism, rheumatoid arthritis, primary amyloidosis and kidney failure (Yonuki et al, 2017).

Hannan and Sawaya (2001) also point out that one of the main causes of median nerve entrapment is repetitive wrist movements, such as knitting, typing on a keyboard, scrubbing, washing clothes, driving, painting and gardening. Still on the subject of triggering factors, Ashworth (2009) points out that most causes are difficult to identify (idiopathic causes). However, he points to some secondary causes, such as space-occupying lesions like tumors, synovial tissue hypertrophy, the formation of bone callus after fractures and osteophytes, metabolic and physiological changes, hypothyroidism, pregnancy, rheumatoid arthritis), infections, neuropathies associated with diabetes or alcoholism and rheumatic changes. Mechanical causes are also mentioned, such as repetitive activities requiring wrist flexion and extension, obesity, hysterectomy without oophorectomy and recent menopause.

1.1.3. Treatment

Based on the literature consulted and according to the existing guidelines for carpal tunnel syndrome, treatment should be started at an early stage and should consist of conservative treatment if there are no signs of median nerve atrophy yet, as observed by electromyography (Hadianfard et al, 2015). According to

According to the authors, conservative treatment includes immobilization with a wrist splint, local corticosteroid injections and daily forearm and wrist strengthening exercises. Surgery is recommended if conservative treatment fails to significantly improve symptoms.

For Yonuki and colleagues (2017), and as observed in the rest of the literature, treatment is divided into surgical and non-surgical, with non-surgical treatment including the placement of a splint to reduce wrist movement and the use of corticosteroids, either orally or by local injection. During the night, the use of a splint also aims to avoid prolonged periods of excessive wrist flexion during sleep. In addition to these aspects, the authors also mention the existence of other available options, namely the use of vit. B6 and B12, non-steroidal anti-inflammatory drugs and exercise, among others.

Surgical treatment is divided into open surgery and endoscopic surgery, the former requiring a longer recovery time for the patient and the existence of a scar, which can alter the patient's level of satisfaction. The latter, on the other hand, has a shorter recovery time and the formation of scar tissue, but an increased risk of nerve or artery damage due to the difficulty in visualizing the structures properly. Thus, in the opinion of the authors, the choice of method varies depending on the surgeon's experience and the user's preference (yonuki et al, 2017).

However, surgical results do not always provide an adequate and satisfactory response to the problem. Gurcay et al. (2016) carried out a study comparing the effect of local corticoid injection and decompressive surgery and concluded that the two methods showed clinical improvement and electrophysiological parameters, with no short-term improvement of one approach over the other, and no statistically significant differences were found with regard to pain, weakness and tingling.

Kim and colleagues (2016) also used the Boston questionnaire to assess the symptoms of CCS at various times, namely preoperatively, in the immediate postoperative period, 2 weeks after surgery and 12 weeks after surgery, and found that there was an improvement in symptoms 2 weeks after surgery, while functionality improved only after 12 weeks, which limits user satisfaction. Thus, the authors concluded that surgery quickly resolves clinical symptoms, but median nerve edema and hand function take several months to improve.

Effectiveness of acupuncture in controlling the symptoms of Carpal Canal Syndrome

Bland and colleagues (2007) emphasize that surgical decompression is considered very effective in many patients, but has varying success rates. This disparity in results is also mentioned by Huisstede and colleagues (2017), who concluded in their study that surgical treatment appears to be more effective than the use of immobilization splints or oral anti-inflammatory drugs, in combination with other hand therapies, in the short, medium and long term for treating CCS. However, there is strong evidence that local corticosteroid injection is more effective than surgery in the short term, and moderate evidence that manual therapy is more effective than surgery in the short and medium term. There is no unequivocal evidence to suggest that one surgical treatment is more effective than the other.

Faced with this difficulty in pinpointing the best therapeutic approach for curing CCS through the literature found, and as a way of reinforcing the existing literature, Wipperman and Goerl (2016) point out that conservative treatment can first be presented to the patient if the clinical picture is mild to moderate. Therapeutic options include immobilization with a splint, corticosteroids, physical exercise to strengthen muscles, ultrasound and yoga. According to these authors, the injection of local corticosteroids produces relief for more than a month and can delay the need for surgery by up to a year. If the patient has severe carpal tunnel syndrome, with no relief from symptoms with conservative treatment, surgical decompression should be performed.

Regarding the use of the immobilization splint, Nobuta et al. (2017) advise their users to wear it at night, reserving its use during the day only when symptoms are more pronounced. However, the length of time the splint should be worn is also controversial, as according to Walker et al. (2000) the effectiveness is much higher when the user wears the splint continuously, compared to wearing it only at night.

For Yunoki et al. (2017), surgery is only indicated when there are very significant sensory changes, and in their study, of the 29 patients who underwent surgery, 13 were in stage 3, with imminent atrophy of the tenar muscle.

In an attempt to understand the best therapeutic approach for treating CCS, Ashworth (2009) carried out a systematic review of the literature, which covered the following therapeutic approaches: acupuncture, open or endoscopic surgery, the use of medication such as diuretics, systemic or local corticosteroids, massage therapy, therapeutic exercises, non-steroidal anti-inflammatory drugs, pyridoxine, ultrasound and the use of an immobilization splint. The results showed some benefits in terms of symptom reduction with some therapeutic approaches, but there is still no 100% effective answer to solving this health problem. The author also found no studies that consistently prove the benefits of acupuncture in controlling the symptoms of this pathology.

As can be seen from the literature found, there is still no treatment that guarantees a complete and definitive recovery, so there is an urgent need to find complementary and multidisciplinary alternatives that improve the range of therapeutic options and consequently the quality of life of patients with CCS, *considering the important role that could be played by traditional Chinese medicine (TCM), and in particular acupuncture, in patients with CCS without surgical indication and in the pre- and post-operative approach in the case of patients with surgical indication.*

2. TRADITIONAL CHINESE MEDICINE

Traditional Chinese Medicine (TCM) began, in Greten's opinion (2008), with the appearance of the book "Yellow Emperor's Classic on Internal Medicine", some 2300 years ago. This book is presented in the form of a dialogue between Huang Di, the Yellow Emperor and his doctor, Chi Po. The Emperor asks questions about health and the causes and treatment of illnesses and Chi Po explains to the Emperor the principles of healthy living in order to achieve longevity. He discusses the functions of the various organ systems, the meridians and their harmonious interaction when we are healthy, as well as the changes that occur when we are ill (Stux & Pomeranz, 1987).

According to Porkert (1974), traditional Chinese medicine is a highly theoretical and abstract doctrine, based on concepts such as Yin and Yang, with acupuncture emerging as an empirical science that emerged from the discovery that needles placed in the skin produce effects on certain organs, usually at some distance from where they were placed, even on organs that, in the light of modern anatomy, do not exist. TCM is based on the theory of Yin and Yang, which correspond to structure and activity, respectively, thus constituting opposite poles of polarity and directionality (Porkert, 2001). Stux and Pomeranz (1987) point out that all opposites in nature develop within this field of tension between Yin and Yang, which constitute a dynamic polarity between them, complementing each other. They thus create a dynamic process, one of which cannot exist without the other. In this way, Yang is the sky, Yin is the earth; Yang is the male, Yin is the female; Yang is hot, Yin is cold; Yang is active, Yin is passive.

The same authors state that the universe is seen as a complex network of highly related processes, carried out by opposing forces, which always combine to make up the whole (Yin cannot exist without Yang and vice versa). Thus, we can say that TCM is based on the theory of Yin and Yang, which correspond to structure and function, respectively, thus constituting opposite poles of polarity and directionality (Porkert, 2001).

Quoting Yong Yan and collaborators (2006), TCM is an integrative medicine that contains science, humanism and characteristics of Chinese culture. The same authors also point out that it is based on a basic theory that emphasizes humanism, argues that the human body is an organic entity, and that the changes that occur in humans depend on the natural environment that surrounds them.

It is within this more humanistic line of thought that Greten (2008) states that TCM can be characterized by the binomial Yin and Yang and by the natural elements, wood, fire, earth, water and metal, which influence human functioning, stressing, however, that the reading of this interaction must be done with the heart. These elements or evolutionary phases are related to certain areas/functions of the human body called orbs, which are considered clinical manifestations of a phase. A group of diagnostically relevant signs, indicating the functional state of a body island (body region), which correlates with the functional properties of a conduit, (Greten, 2006). Thus, the "wood" evolutionary phase corresponds to manifestations in the liver orb, the "fire" evolutionary phase corresponds to the heart orb, the "earth" evolutionary phase to the orb corresponding to the Spleen Pancreas and the stomach, the "metal" evolutionary phase to the lung orb and the "water" evolutionary phase to the kidney orb.

2.1. Diagnosis in TCM

In addition to these assumptions, TCM is based on the ability to determine the Chinese diagnosis. This, according to Porkert (2001) and Greten (2008), is made up of 4 parts, namely the constitution, the agent, the orb and the guiding criteria, which allow us to determine the appropriate treatment for the patient.

The **constitution** is the part of the diagnosis that defines the internal nature of the patient through the expression of their physical appearance. This shows that Chinese medicine believes that physical structure modifies an individual's functional behavior, therefore their feelings, functions and the likelihood of certain symptoms (Greten, 2008).

The **agent** is the pathogenic factor, i.e. the cause of the disease. In Chinese medicine, pathogenic factors are all factors that interfere with or disturb the normal flow of the individual's energy (Hempen & Chow, 2006). These agents are divided into 3 groups, depending on their origin. Thus, we have external or exogenous factors, metaphorically referred to as the six climatic excesses, corresponding the neurovegetative reaction observed to that which occurs when an individual is exposed to these climatic agents: wind (ventus), cold (*algor*), heat (calor), aestus (golpe de sol), humidity (humor), ariditas (prolonged exposure to dryness) and ardor (ardor) (Porkert, 2001; Greten, 2008; Hempen & Chow, 2006). With regard to internal agents, the same authors point to the seven primordial emotions as the main ones. Internal agents can induce alterations or deviations in the normal flow of neurovegetative regulation and functional capacity, often referred to as energy. Thus, the internal agents are: *voluptas* (excessive manifestation of joy, will and pleasure), anger and excessive impulsivity, anxiety (*Timor*), sadness (*maeror*), fear and obsessive thoughts (*cogitatio*), dread and solicitude. Neutral agents are: overwork, eating disorders, excessive alcohol, excessive sexual activity, trauma, infections, excessive stress, etc. (Porkert, 2001; Greten, 2008; Hempen & Chow, 2006).

The **orb** is the third main constituent of the Chinese diagnosis. This word refers to the Latin word "orbis" which means circle. It is a circle or group of diagnostically significant signs and findings that are grouped and named according to organs or regions where some of the symptoms occur. This is sometimes referred to as the Chinese doctrine of the organs, which is a simplified understanding of the system and used differently from Western medicine (Greten, 2008).

The fourth step of Chinese diagnosis is made up of the eight **guiding criteria**. These constitute the basic and essential condition for any diagnosis, as a way of providing consistency and making any treatment effective (Porkert, 2001). The same author states that the eight guiding criteria correspond to four pairs of polar qualities, namely *repletion* and *depletion*, *heat and heat, extima and intima and Yin* and *Yang.*

Greten (2008) points out that a guiding criterion can be understood as the evaluation of clinical signs according to an underlying model of physiological regulation.

The same author mentions that the first guiding criterion is called **repletion/depletion,** pointing out that it assesses clinical signs that traditional Chinese medicine believes originate from *qi* and the *orbs.* Thus, *repletion* indicates the presence of too much qi in the body, which in turn causes certain symptoms. In turn, signs of *depletion* indicate a lack of qi in the body. Porkert (2001) also states that *depletion* corresponds to a deficiency of content, or to be more precise, an imperfect filling of the body's resources and potentials.

The second guiding criterion is called **heat/heat** and, according to Greten (2008), evaluates signs that for TCM originate in the effects of *xue* (blood and its functions), which is the second functional power or source of energy in Chinese medicine. Thus, signs of xue hyperactivation correspond to hyperstimulation of the microcirculation and correspond to the heat guide criterion; on the other hand, signs of decreased microcirculation functions correspond to the *algorithm* guide criterion.

With regard to this guiding criterion, Porkert (2001) points out that *algorithm* denotes a decrease in functions, activity, metabolism and consequently a decrease in vital heat. In contrast, heat corresponds to an acceleration of vital functions, activity, reactions and metabolism, which leads to an increase in body temperature, the consequences of which are an increase in the evaporation and dispersion of liquids, which is associated with a loss of body substance.

We now turn to the third guiding criterion, called **extima/intima,** which corresponds to the effect caused by the external agent when it invades the body from the outside in. According to Greten (2008), Chinese medicine presents an explanatory model for the appearance and progression of disease, based on the pathophysiological model of the six stages of cold invasion (algor) called Algor Laedens Theory, or "the doctrine of cold invading the body".

For Porkert (2001), the *extima* corresponds to the body surface, including the skin, the hair and the arteries found in the skin. Thus, for this author, changes in the *extima* are accessible to sensory perception and mechanical action. In contrast, changes to the *intima* affect the body's internal organs, leading over time to serious and chronic illnesses, particularly if the body's defenses (immune system) are weakened.

Finally, the fourth guiding criterion, **Yin/Yang,** corresponds to the structure versus function of the organism. Greten (2008) points out that this guiding criterion evaluates signs which, in the light of TCM, distinguish between a primary, more functional dysregulation (yang) and a secondary dysregulation due to a structural deficiency (yin).

In this sense, Greten (2008) points out that TCM is based on a system that describes functional abnormalities through their signs and symptoms, i.e. a system of sensations and discoveries aimed at establishing a functional vegetative state. This state can be treated with phytopharmacology, acupuncture, Chinese manual therapy (Tuina), Qi Gong or dietetics.

2.2. Traditional Chinese Medicine and pain

TCM has a number of techniques that have proven to be very effective in controlling pain, namely Tuina massage, which is short for Chinese Manual Therapy, and acupuncture. As described above, diagnosis in TCM is understood as an assessment of the body's vegetative functional state, based on which an appropriate set of acupoints is selected, which have certain functions and clinical effects, being connected to deeper layers of the body, influencing the circulation of "Qi". These same points can be stimulated through the introduction of acupuncture needles or through Tuina massage techniques (Sousa et al, 2015). Thus, we can say that Tuina massage incorporates several principles of acupuncture, including the use of acupoints, through which it is possible to remove energy blockages along the affected conduits.

According to TCM, the state of health reflects a basic state of balance of Qi and blood in the human body. Qi can be understood as the "neurovegetative capacity of an organ or tissue to function, presenting itself sensorially as a sensation of tearing, pressure or flow" (Greten, 2013). In this sense, Yang and collaborators (2014) reinforce that pain is usually caused by the obstruction of Qi and consequently by the obstruction of blood circulation in the affected body region. The same authors point out that pathogenic factors such as blood stasis, Qi stasis, dampness, phlegm and others can be identified as causes of blockages. As a way of highlighting these assumptions, we quote Ernst (2006) who states that in TCM philosophy, health is considered to be the balance between two complementary opposite poles, yin and yang, which correspond, in the light of conventional medicine, to the sympathetic nervous system and the parasympathetic nervous system, respectively. Diseases are associated with an imbalance which, as mentioned above, is commonly related to disturbances in the circulation of Qi, and TCM's main objective is to remove such disturbances.

2.2.1. Tuina massage and pain

The main aim of Tuina massage is to remove the energy blockages that lead to Qi stagnation. This massage will increase the circulation of Qi and blood and reduce localized edema, which in turn will help to reduce pain. The painful spot is usually where the energy and blood blockage is located. Thus, manipulating these points will move the blockages in order to promote the free circulation of Qi and increase blood circulation in the affected area, (Yang et al, 2014). These authors point to studies that have shown that one of the mechanisms through which Tuina massage appears to be beneficial is in reducing inflammation and promoting mitochondrial biogenesis, which leads to the repair of damaged skeletal muscle tissue.

Tuina massage, whose original name is "tui na an mo", is made up of more than 50 classic forms of manipulation and four components that can be mixed with these techniques: pressure, vibration, movement and heating.

Sousa and colleagues (2015) point out that several studies show the effectiveness of Tuina in different clinical situations, such as stress and anxiety, neck stiffness, low back pain, pain caused by herniated discs and others.

Jiang et al. (2016) also confirmed these conclusions in their randomized study, in which they brought together 98 individuals with Carpal Canal Syndrome who were divided into two groups, a treatment group and a control group. The treatment group received acupuncture at specifically selected points, followed by Tuina relaxation massage. The control group received conventional pharmacological treatment. The results obtained showed a statistically significant difference between the two groups (P<0.01), with the percentage of cure being 81.7% for the treatment group and 47.4% for the control group, which leads to the conclusion that acupuncture in conjunction with Tuina massage are a simple therapy, but with considerable effects for carpal tunnel syndrome.

However, based on the literature consulted, we found that its effectiveness has already been demonstrated in the management of various pathologies, such as major depressive syndromes, substance abuse and addiction, immune and autoimmune diseases, failure to respond to therapy in premature infants and pain syndromes, particularly musculoskeletal disorders (Kumar et al, 2013).

Also with the aim of demonstrating the effectiveness of Tuina massage in reducing pain, we highlight the findings of Lewis and Johnson (2006), who evaluated 20 studies that included a total of 1,341 participants, with the aim of investigating the effect of Tuina massage on pain control. 9 of these studies were carried out on healthy individuals, and the interventions were carried out with the aim of reducing post-exercise pain; 11 studies were carried out on patients with musculoskeletal diseases whose symptoms included the presence of pain. Massage therapy proved to be effective in reducing pain in half of these 20 studies, and of the 9 studies carried out on healthy individuals, 4 showed an improvement in their pain. In the group of patients with musculoskeletal disorders, 6 also showed positive results when compared to the control group. However, the authors point out that the small size of the samples, the methodological quality of the studies and the short duration of the massage mean that the results are inconclusive.

Tsao (2007) also carried out a systematic review of the literature and found that

patients with CFS who received Tuina massage for a period of 4 weeks, 15 minutes a day, showed an improvement in pain, grip strength, anxiety and depression when compared to the control group.

2.2.2. Acupuncture and pain

Acupuncture is already widely known in the Western world and is widely referenced in international literature. It represents a part of traditional Chinese medicine and is included in holistic therapies, since the diagnosis is not based on radiological and laboratory tests, but on the sensory organs of the therapists and the subjective sensations reported by the patients, which leads to a personalized diagnosis and treatment, (Kubiena & Sommer, 2010).

The same authors also point out that the way it works is based on the premise that by inserting needles into certain acupuncture points on the human body, they trigger not only a local effect, but also a systemic effect, since they produce mobilization of vital energy, Qi, which restores balance, drains excess and eliminates stagnation. In this sense, Hempen and Chow (2006) state that acupuncture is the method of treating health problems by inserting needles into certain points on the human body for therapeutic purposes.

According to Greten (2015), there are 4 basic pathogenic mechanisms: problems in transmission between phases; excess of an agent; disturbance of an antagonist; and yin deficiency. Thus, we can say that, with regard to the problem of transmission between phases, the movement started in one phase must continue to the next phase and so on. However, this mechanism generally fails due to insufficient Earth orbs (stomach and spleen/pancreas), which leads to a blockage. Regarding the excess of an agent, Greten (2015) points out that there are several agents that can cause disturbances in this transition between phases, namely external agents (algorithm, wind, mood...); internal agents (emotions); and neutral agents (stress, pollution, etc.). With regard to the disturbance of an antagonist, one of the main changes observed is the **Wood-Metal** imbalance, i.e. based on the characteristics of the liver orb: full chest, clenched fists, hypertonic muscles, strong and loud voice, which shows a lack of relaxation, which is on the same axis as the pulmonary orb whose characteristics are small chest, flaccid hands, flaccid muscles and low voice, it is easy to see the difficulty in maintaining this balance, taking into account the

overlapping of the liver orb over the lung orb, which is weak by constitution. The last disease mechanism is yin deficiency. This deficiency can be understood as a decrease in body structure, which causes morphological changes that, together with bodily and neurological dysfunctions, lead to the appearance of pain (Greten, 2015).

Based on the knowledge that acupuncture's main mechanism of action is the removal of energy blockages and, consequently, the improvement of Qi and blood circulation, it is easy to see that one of its main therapeutic indications is analgesia. Stux and Pomeranz (1987) point out that acupuncture activates small nerve fibers centered in the muscles, which send impulses to the spinal cord, which in turn activates 3 important centers, the spinal cord, midbrain and pituitary-hypothalamus, which release endorphins that cause analgesia.

Naslund and Odenbring (2002) argue that the physiological response of acupuncture in the human body occurs at three levels: the local effect, which arises when an acupuncture point is stimulated through the insertion of a needle; the effect on the spinal cord, which occurs after the insertion of the needle and is linked to the release of neuropeptides into the cerebrospinal fluid; and finally, the effect at the cortical level, with the release of endorphins and serotonin.

Thus, based on the mechanisms mentioned above, Stux and Pomeranz (1987), based on various studies, concluded that, with regard to analgesia, acupuncture is very effective in the treatment of chronic pain, helping 55 to 85% of patients, with favorable results for acupuncture when compared to the use of analgesic medication (for example, morphine helps in 70% of cases). In addition, they concluded that acupuncture is more effective than placebo, indicating a real physical effect.

2.2.3. Acupuncture and carpal tunnel syndrome

Acupuncture as a therapeutic intervention is widely practiced. Although there are many studies on its potential usefulness, many of these studies provide dubious results due to the methodology used, sample size and other factors. However, some promising results have emerged in recent years, showing the effectiveness of acupuncture in the case of nausea and vomiting after surgery or in the case of adult chemotherapy and in post-operative dental pain. There are also other situations, such as in cases of addiction, stroke rehabilitation, headache, menstrual cramps, tennis elbow, fibromyalgia, myofascial pain, osteoarthritis, low back pain, **carpal tunnel syndrome** and asthma, in which acupuncture can be useful as a complementary treatment or an acceptable alternative in recovery programs for individuals (NIH Consenus Conference, 1998).

With regard to the treatment of carpal tunnel syndrome, there is also a large body of literature demonstrating that it is effective in controlling the symptoms associated with this condition. Hadianfard et al. (2014) carried out a randomized study with a sample of 50 patients in which they compared the various therapeutic options for carpal tunnel syndrome and found that patients who underwent acupuncture obtained better results in terms of pain reduction than those who used ibuprofen. In addition to pain, they also obtained better results in terms of improving the sensation of tingling and numbness. The group of patients who received acupuncture also had better results in terms of the frequency with which they woke up at night as a result of pain or other symptoms related to the condition under study.

Another study showing positive results from the use of acupuncture in carpal tunnel syndrome was carried out by Ho Cy and colleagues (2014) who concluded that acupuncture had a positive therapeutic effect, namely improving symptoms, increasing grip strength and electrophysiological function.

Evidence of the effect of acupuncture on improving symptoms in carpal tunnel syndrome was also reported by Prime and colleagues (2010) when they found that among the non-pharmacological approaches, acupuncture showed a significant improvement in median nerve function when compared to other non-pharmacological approaches.

Yang et al. (2009) also compared the effect of acupuncture, using the Pericardium 5 and Pericardium 6 points in the treatment of CCS, with the use of oral prednisolone and found that at the end of the treatment period the improvements were identical in both groups, with the exception of the symptom "waking up during the night as a result of symptoms" which showed more significant results in the group that underwent acupuncture.

In this respect, De-feng (2010) carried out a study to investigate the effectiveness of acupuncture and Tuina massage in 98 patients with CFS and found that acupuncture together with Tuina manipulation had very significant therapeutic effects.

In 2010, Carlson and colleagues looked at the various non-surgical therapeutic alternatives for controlling symptoms of CFS and found that 38% of the American population used so-called *complementary therapies to* control pain.

On this subject, Branco and Naeser (1999) carried out a study using various non-pharmacological approaches, including acupuncture and laser, and found a complete reduction in pain of 50%, and in the follow-up after 1 to 2 years, of the 23 hands treated, only 2 (8.3%) had a recurrence of pain, which quickly reversed after a few weeks of treatment. The same authors found that these results are related to an increase in blood circulation to the brain, particularly to the thalamus. They also point to an increase in adenosine triphosphate (ATP) at cellular level, a reduction in inflammation and a temporary increase in serotonin as possible mechanisms.

We also quote Chung et al. (2016) who state in the literature review carried out for their study that acupuncture is widely used in the treatment of pain and neuropathy in Chinese medicine. The same authors present the results of a systematic review of the literature carried out in 2011, which included two studies comparing acupuncture with local steroid injection and found that the group that underwent acupuncture treatment showed more significant improvements in symptom reduction in carpal tunnel syndrome, compared to the group that underwent injectable corticosteroids. They also highlight another randomized study published in 2009 which showed that patients who received acupuncture treatment showed more significant improvements than patients who took low doses of oral corticosteroids.

Confirming these results, Khosrawi et al. (2012) carried out a randomized controlled study with the aim of verifying the effectiveness of acupuncture in the treatment of mild to moderate symptoms of carpal tunnel syndrome, in which patients underwent 8 sessions of acupuncture compared to the control group who underwent 4 weeks of nocturnal immobilization of the hand, the administration of vit. The authors concluded that acupuncture can improve subjective symptoms in general and can be included in the care programs of these patients. The acupuncture points selected by the aforementioned authors were Pc 7 and Pc 6.

In conclusion, and in order to confirm the long way to go in this area, we quote these authors, who state that in 2010 a systematic review of the literature was carried out to assess the effectiveness of acupuncture in the treatment of CCS, which concluded that the existing findings are not yet convincing enough to suggest that acupuncture is an effective therapy for the treatment of this pathology. However, the National Institute of Health (NIH) has confirmed acupuncture for the management of mild to moderate CCS, although its effectiveness is still controversial (Khosrawi et al.; 2012).

3. METHODOLOGY

In this chapter, we present a set of steps that enabled us to achieve the objectives proposed during the course of this study. According to Fortin (2009), the methodological phase refers to all the means and activities required to answer the research questions or to verify the hypotheses formulated during the conceptual phase.

3.1. Objective of the study

The main objective of this study was to **evaluate the effectiveness of acupuncture in the treatment of Canai Càrpico Syndrome.**

3.2. Type of study

This is a descriptive study because, as Fortin (2009) points out, it aims to identify the characteristics of a phenomenon in order to obtain an overview of a situation or a population. Among the descriptive studies is the case study. This consists of a detailed and complete examination of a phenomenon linked to a social entity (individual, family, community or organization) (Fortin, 2009). Based on this point of view, we can consider that patients with Carpal Canal Syndrome are a group that this study will focus on. According to Fortin (2009, p.241), *a case study can be used to verify the effectiveness of a treatment, to increase our knowledge of an individual or a group and formulate hypotheses for this purpose, or to study the changes likely to occur over time in the individual or group.*

Despite the small sample size, which gives case studies a lack of scientific rigor, Yin (2003) cited by Fortin (2009, 242) *points out that case studies have real scientific value because, among other things, of the in-depth nature of the analysis and the multiple observations they give rise to.*

The sample was selected from patients who had undergone treatment at Clinica Carlos Cotrim II - Cuidados de Saùde, Lda, and who voluntarily agreed to take part in the study.

3.3. Instruments used

The instrument selected was the Boston Questionnaire, which is a self-assessment test consisting of a set of questions that assess the severity of symptoms and the patient's functional status at the time of application.

The version used in this study was translated and validated into Brazilian Portuguese by Campos et al. in 2003, as can be seen in Table 1. In the opinion of the authors, the translation and adaptation of the questionnaire did not pose any difficulties, as it was a simple questionnaire, with questions covering usual symptoms and activities commonly carried out by the general population (Campos et al, 2003).

This questionnaire is self-administered and consists of two scales that assess the severity of symptoms and the functional status of patients with carpal tunnel syndrome. The symptom severity scale assesses symptoms in terms of severity, frequency, timing and type. The functional status scale assesses how the syndrome affects daily life (Meirelles et al, 2006).

The same authors state that the symptom severity scale consists of 11 questions which assess: the intensity of pain during the day and night; frequency of pain during the day and night; duration of pain during the day and night; numbness, weakness, presence of tingling, frequency of tingling during the night and weakness. Each question has five answers, numbered from 1 to 5 and placed in ascending order of symptom severity. Thus, 1 indicates no symptom, 2 little symptom, 3 moderate symptom, 4 intense symptom and 5 indicates severe symptom.

The functional status assessment scale consists of eight questions, which correspond to functional activities such as writing, buttoning clothes, holding a book while reading, holding the telephone, housework, opening the lid of a bottle, carrying shopping bags, bathing and dressing. Each activity has 5 levels of difficulty, with level 1 corresponding to no difficulty, level 2 to little difficulty, level 3 to moderate difficulty, level 4 to intense difficulty and level 5 to being unable to perform the task due to symptoms in the hands and wrists (Meirelles et al, 2006). In addition to the scales presented, the grip strength of the affected hand was also assessed before and after treatment using a dynamometer.

TABLE 1: Self-assessment protocol - Boston Questionnaire (Source: Meirelles et al, 2006).

SELF-ASSESSMENT PROTOCOL - BOSTON PROTOCOL

Name: Hand: ( ) Right ( ) Left Date of evaluation: ..../......./........

THE FOLLOWING QUESTIONS REFER TO YOUR

SYMPTOMS IN A TYPICAL 24-HOUR PERIOD,

DURING THE LAST TWO WEEKS.

(Check one answer for each question)

1) How severe is the pain in your hand or wrist at night?

1. I have no pain in my hand or wrist at night

2. little pain

3. moderate pain

4. severe pain

5. very intense pain

2) How many times has pain in your hand or wrist woken you up during a typical night in the last two weeks?

1. none

2. a

3. two to three times

4. four to five times

5. more than five times

3) Do you usually have pain in your hand or wrist during the day?

1. I never have pain during the day

2. I have little pain during the day

3. I have moderate pain during the day

4. I have intense pain during the day

5. I have very intense pain during the day

4) How often do you get pain in your hand or wrist during the day?

1. never

2. once or twice a day

3. three to five times a day

4. more than five times a day

5. the pain is constant

5) How long, on average, do pain episodes last during the day?

1. I never have pain during the day

2. less than 10 minutes

3. from 10 to 60 minutes

4. more than 60 minutes

5. the pain is constant during the day

6) Do you have numbness (loss of feeling) in your hand?

1. no

2. I have little sleep

3. I have moderate numbness

4. I have intense numbness

5. I have very intense numbness

7) Do you have weakness in your hand or wrist?

1. no weakness

2. little weakness

3. moderate weakness

4. intense weakness

5. very intense weakness

8) Do you feel a tingling sensation in your hand?

1. no tingling

2. little tingling

3. moderate tingling

4. intense tingling

5. very intense tingling

9) How intense is the numbness (loss of feeling) or tingling at night?

1. I don't feel numb or tingly at night

2. little

3. moderate

4. intense

5. very intense

10) How often has numbness or tingling woken you up during a typical night in the last two weeks?

1. none

2. a

3. two to three times

4. four to five times

5. very intense

11) Do you have difficulty picking up and using small objects, such as keys or pens?

1. without difficulty

2. little difficulty

3. moderate difficulty

4. intense difficulty

5. very intense difficulty

ON A TYPICAL DAY, DURING THE LAST TWO WEEKS, HAVE YOUR HAND OR WRIST SYMPTOMS CAUSED YOU ANY DIFFICULTY IN DOING THE ACTIVITIES LISTED BELOW?

Please circle the number that best describes your ability to do each activity

ACTIVITY	GRADE OF
Writing	DIFFICULTY
	1 2 3 4 5
Buttoning clothes	1 2 3 4 5
Holding a book while reading	1 2 3 4 5
Holding the phone	1 2 3 4 5
Housework	1 2 3 4 5
Opening a bottle cap	1 2 3 4 5
Carrying grocery bags	1 2 3 4 5
Bathing and dressing	1 2 3 4 5

No difficulty 1

Little difficulty 2

Moderate difficulty 3

Intense difficulty 4

Can't do any work at all because of hand and wrist symptoms 5

Observer's opinion: ____

3.4. Procedures

Acupuncture was performed with disposable, single-use, stainless steel needles measuring 0.25x40 mm. The skin at the puncture site was disinfected with 70° alcohol. The depth of the puncture and the intensity of the stimulation produced by the needle were maintained. The needles remained in place for a period of 40 minutes and the sessions were carried out twice a week over a period of 6 weeks. All the needles were inserted to a depth of about 0.5 *cun* (the cun is a unit of measurement centered on the patient, corresponding to the distance between the distal and proximal part of the interphalangeal joint of the thumb, Kubiena & Sommer, 2008).

The selection of points was based on the symptoms presented by the patients and the therapeutic indications for each point. The acupuncture points selected for this study were Pericardium 6 (Pc 6), Tricaloric 4 (Tc 4) and Tricaloric 5 (Tc 5).

Pericardium 6 (Pc 6): Internal Clusa

This point is located in the pericardial conduit, 2 *cun* (the standardized measurement used in TCM) above the transverse line of the wrist, on the anterior surface of the hand, between the *palmaris longus* and *flexor carpi radialis* tendons. In the opinion of Greten (2008) this point, although it doesn't belong to the 5 ancient points, is particularly important because it is the nexus of the pericardial conduit. In other words, it connects the pericardial conduit with the tricaloric conduit via Tc 5, which is located on the opposite side of the arm. In addition, it is a connection point with the *yin retaining synerarchy, which means that* it has a strong harmonizing effect, as it connects all the yin orbs and all the yin conduits in the body.

The pericardial conduit is indicated for symptoms such as pain, alterations in sensitivity and muscle control, as well as for skin disorders that lie along the path of this meridian (Porkert, 1995). The same author lists a wide range of therapeutic indications for this point, highlighting pain in the wrist, elbow and/or the entire upper limb; tension or spasms affecting the upper limbs and neck stiffness.

Hempen and Chow (2006) also point out that the main therapeutic indications are wrist pain, tension in the upper extremities, among others. For these reasons, this was one of the points selected for the treatment of carpal tunnel syndrome.

Tricaloric 4 (Tc 4): Stagnum Yang

This conduit also has therapeutic indications for pain control and changes in sensitivity and muscle control, as well as skin disorders along the conduit (Porkert, 1995).

The Stagnum Yang point is located in the depression between the ulna and the metacarpal bone, lateral to the *extensor digitorum* tendon and its main indications are wrist pain, pain and stiffness in the arm and shoulders, among others (Hempen & Chow, 2006; Porkert, 1995). The choice of this point is based on these therapeutic indications.

Tricaloric 5 (Tc 5): External Cluse

As part of the conduit described above, the external clusa point is located 2 *cun* above the midline of the wrist, on the back of the arm, between the radius and the ulna. This point activates the *retaining yang artery* and its main effect is to free the conduits from existing narrowings (Greten, 2008). The same author also points out that the tricaloric conduit frees the passage of water and mobilizes Qi, fluids and blood (xue), thus eliminating Qi blockages.

The main indications for the Tc 5 point are pain, weakness and paresthesia in the fingers and elbow pain. These indications justify its choice in the treatment of carpal tunnel syndrome, since one of the characteristics of the disease is pain, weakness and paresthesia of the fingers of the hand (Hempen & Chow, 2006; Porkert, 1995).

3L5L **Ethical Considerations**

The elaboration of any research implies, most of the time, the raising of ethical and moral questions. According to Streubert and Carpenter (2002, p.67), *ethical considerations are and always will be critical. Committing to a research study implies a personal and professional responsibility to ensure that the design of quantitative or qualitative studies is ethically and morally sound.*

As far as the current study is concerned, we would like to highlight the fact that it focused on an autonomous population, taking into account that all the participants were of legal age. In addition to this, the protection of anonymity and data confidentiality was guaranteed. Participants were also guaranteed total respect for their wishes if they decided not to take part in the study, and no harm would come to them as a result.

An informed consent form was signed. According to Fortin (1999), the consent form is a document in which the subject declares that they have been well informed about the research project and that they agree to take part in it, autonomously and voluntarily.

3.6. Presentation of Clinical Cases

Case 1: A 38-year-old woman, a dental assistant, complained of intense and continuous pain in both hands and wrists for about 15 months. A medical diagnosis of carpal tunnel syndrome was made around 10 months ago; she has undergone various pharmacological treatments to reduce symptoms, including analgesia and local corticosteroid injections. To achieve a reduction in symptoms, he also resorted, on medical advice, to immobilization through the use of a splint at night and, during the most symptomatic periods, also during the day. None of these approaches worked, so surgical intervention was planned. 3 days before her anesthesiology appointment, she came to my office to ask for an opinion and had her first acupuncture treatment. According to the patient, there was an immediate 70% reduction in symptoms. She cancelled her anesthesiology appointment by phone and had twice-weekly treatments for 6 weeks. The symptoms regressed completely, as can be seen from the answers given in the Boston questionnaire (Tables 2 and 3).

The patient said that before the treatment she was no longer able to carry out a large number of daily activities, such as opening the door or holding her 5-year-old son. After 6 weeks of treatment, the symptoms completely regressed and did not interfere with her daily life.

Before the acupuncture treatment: right hand: 10 kg; left hand: 8 kg. After the 6-week treatment: right hand: 40 kg; left hand: 35 kg.

TABLE 2: Boston Questionnaire, clinical case 1, before the start of treatment

SELF-ASSESSMENT PROTOCOL - PROTOCOL

FROM BOSTON

Name: V. A.

Hand: (x) Right (x) Left

Evaluation date: **1/6/2017**

THE FOLLOWING QUESTIONS REFER TO YOUR

SYMPTOMS IN A TYPICAL 24-HOUR PERIOD,

DURING THE LAST TWO WEEKS.

(Check one answer for each question)

1) How severe is the pain in your hand or wrist at night?

1. I have no pain in my hand or wrist at night

2. little pain

3. moderate pain

X 4. severe pain

5. very intense pain

2) How many times has pain in your hand or wrist woken you up during a typical night in the last two weeks?

1. none

2. a

X 3. two to three times

4. four to five times

5. more than five times

3) Do you usually have pain in your hand or wrist during the day?

1. I never have pain during the day

2. I have little pain during the day

3. I have moderate pain during the day

4. I have intense pain during the day

X 5. I have very intense pain during the day

4) How often do you get pain in your hand or wrist during the day?

1. never

2. once or twice a day

3. three to five times a day

4. more than five times a day

X 5. pain is constant

5) How long, on average, do pain episodes last during the day?

1. I never have pain during the day

2. less than 10 minutes

3. from 10 to 60 minutes

4. more than 60 minutes

X 5. the pain is constant during the day

6) Do you have numbness (loss of feeling) in your hand?

1. no

2. I have little sleep

3. I have moderate numbness

4. I have intense numbness

X 5. I have very intense numbness

7) Do you have weakness in your hand or wrist?

1. no weakness

2. little weakness

3. moderate weakness

4. intense weakness

X 5. very intense weakness

8) Do you feel a tingling sensation in your hand?

1. no tingling

2. little tingling

3. moderate tingling

X 4. Intense tingling

No difficulty 1

Little difficulty 2

Moderate difficulty 3

Intense difficulty 4

Can't do any work at all because of hand and wrist symptoms 5

Observer's opinion:

9) How intense is the numbness (loss of feeling) or tingling at night?

1. I don't feel numb or tingly at night

2. little

3. moderate

4. intense

X 5. very intense

10) How often has numbness or tingling woken you up during a typical night in the last two weeks?

1. none

2. a

X 3. two to three times

4. four to five times

5. very intense

11) Do you have difficulty picking up and using small objects, such as keys or pens?

1. without difficulty

2. little difficulty

3. moderate difficulty

X 4. Intense difficulty

5. very intense difficulty

A TYPICAL DAY, DURING THE LAST TWO WEEKS, THE SYMPTOMS OF YOUR HAND OR WRIST HAVE YOU HAD ANY DIFFICULTY DOING THE ACTIVITIES LISTED BELOW?

Please circle the number that best describes your ability to do each activity

ACTIVITY	DEGREE OF DIFFICULTY
Writing	1 2 3 4 **X**

Buttoning clothes	1 2 3 4 **X**
Holding a book while reading	1 2 3 4 **X**
Holding the phone	1 2 3 4 **X**
Housework	1 2 3 4 **X**
Opening a bottle cap	1 2 3 4 **X**
Carrying grocery bags	1 2 3 4 **X**
Bathing and dressing	1 2 3 **X** 5

5. very intense tingling

TABLE 3: Boston Questionnaire, clinical case 1, after 6 weeks of treatment

SELF-ASSESSMENT PROTOCOL - PROTOCOL

FROM BOSTON

Name: V. A.

Hand: (X) Right (X) Left

Date of evaluation: **14/7/2017**

THE FOLLOWING QUESTIONS REFER TO YOUR

SYMPTOMS IN A TYPICAL 24-HOUR PERIOD,

DURING THE LAST TWO WEEKS.

(Check one answer for each question)

1) How severe is the pain in your hand or wrist at night?

X 1. I have no pain in my hand or wrist at night

2. little pain

3. moderate pain

4. severe pain

5. very intense pain

2) How many times has pain in your hand or wrist woken you up during a typical night in the last two weeks?

X 1. none

2. a

3. two to three times

4. four to five times

5. more than five times

3) Do you usually have pain in your hand or wrist during the day?

X 1. I never have pain during the day

2. I have little pain during the day

3. I have moderate pain during the day

4. I have intense pain during the day

5. I have very intense pain during the day

4) How often do you get pain in your hand or wrist during the day?

X 1. never

2. once or twice a day

3. three to five times a day

4. more than five times a day

5. the pain is constant

5) How long, on average, do pain episodes last during the day?

X 1. I never have pain during the day

2. less than 10 minutes

3. from 10 to 60 minutes

4. more than 60 minutes

5. the pain is constant during the day

6) Do you have numbness (loss of feeling) in your hand?

X 1. no

2. I have little sleep

3. I have moderate numbness

4. I have intense numbness

5. I have very intense numbness

7) Do you have weakness in your hand or wrist?

X 1. no weakness

2. little weakness

3. moderate weakness

4. intense weakness

5. very intense weakness

8) Do you feel a tingling sensation in your hand?

X 1. No tingling

2. little tingling

3. moderate tingling

4. intense tingling

5. very intense tingling

9) How intense is the numbness (loss of feeling) or tingling at night?

X 1. I don't feel numb or tingly at night

2. little

3. moderate

4. intense

5. very intense

10) How often has numbness or tingling woken you up during a typical night in the last two weeks?

X 1. none

2. a

3. two to three times

4. four to five times

5. very intense

11) Do you have difficulty picking up and using small objects, such as keys or pens?

X 1. without difficulty

2. little difficulty

3. moderate difficulty

4. intense difficulty

5. very intense difficulty

A TYPICAL DAY, DURING THE LAST TWO

WEEKS, THE SYMPTOMS OF YOUR HAND OR WRIST

HAVE CAUSED HIM SOME DIFFICULTY IN

DO THE ACTIVITIES LISTED BELOW?

Please circle the number that best describes your ability to do each activity

ACTIVITY	DEGREE OF DIFFICULTY			
Writing	**X** 2	3	4	5
Buttoning clothes	**X** 2	3	4	5
Holding a book while reading	**X** 2	3	4	5
Holding the phone	**X** 2	3	4	5
Housework	**X** 2	3	4	5
Opening a bottle cap	**X** 2	3	4	5
Carrying grocery bags	**X** 2	3	4	5
Bathing and dressing	**X** 2	3	4	5

No difficulties 1

Little difficulty 2

Moderate difficulty 3

Intense difficulty 4

Can't do any work at all because of hand and wrist symptoms 5

Observer's opinion:

Case 2: Woman, 52 years old, cleaning lady, complaining of intense pain and tingling in her right hand, several episodes of sick leave due to inability to perform tasks, diagnosed about 2 years ago with carpal tunnel syndrome, underwent several medical interventions without success, was on the waiting list for surgery. She came to my office on the recommendation of a friend and underwent an initial treatment, where she immediately saw a 50-60% improvement. She underwent 6 weeks of twice-weekly treatment, after which her symptoms completely disappeared, as can be seen from her answers to the Boston questionnaire (Charts 4 and 5).

The results obtained were very significant, as in the patient's opinion there was a complete remission of the pain. She does all the household chores without any difficulty and the strength of her grip no longer interferes with her professional life, which was the case before the treatments.

With regard to grip strength, the measurements were: before the start of treatment: Right hand: 8 kg. After the 6-week treatment: Right hand: 25 kg.

TABLE 4: Boston Questionnaire, clinical case 2, before the start of treatment

SELF-ASSESSMENT PROTOCOL - PROTOCOL

FROM BOSTON

Name: R. A.

Hand: (x) Right ( ) Left

Date of evaluation: **28/4/2017**

THE FOLLOWING QUESTIONS REFER TO YOUR

SYMPTOMS IN A TYPICAL 24-HOUR PERIOD,

DURING THE LAST TWO WEEKS.

(Check one answer for each question)

1) How severe is the pain in your hand or wrist at night?

1. I have no pain in my hand or wrist at night

2. little pain

3. moderate pain

X 4. severe pain

5. very intense pain

2) How many times has pain in your hand or wrist woken you up during a typical night in the last two weeks?

1. none

2. a

3. two to three times

X 4. four to five times

5. more than five times

3) Do you usually have pain in your hand or wrist during the day?

1. I never have pain during the day

2. I have little pain during the day

3. I have moderate pain during the day

X 4. I have intense pain during the day

5. I have very intense pain during the day

4) How often do you get pain in your hand or wrist during the day?

1. never

2. once or twice a day

3. three to five times a day

4. more than five times a day

X 5. pain is constant

5) How long, on average, do pain episodes last during the day?

1. I never have pain during the day

2. less than 10 minutes

3. from 10 to 60 minutes

X 4. more than 60 minutes

5. the pain is constant during the day

6) Do you have numbness (loss of feeling) in your hand?

1. no

2. I have little sleep

3. I have moderate numbness

X 4. I have intense numbness

5. I have very intense numbness

7) Do you have weakness in your hand or wrist?

1. no weakness

2. little weakness

3. moderate weakness

X 4. Intense weakness

5. very intense weakness

8) Do you feel a tingling sensation in your hand?

1. no tingling

2. little tingling

3. moderate tingling

X 4. Intense tingling

5. very intense tingling

9) How intense is the numbness (loss of feeling) or tingling at night?

1. I don't feel numb or tingly at night

2. little

3. moderate

X 4. intense

5. very intense

10) How often has numbness or tingling woken you up during a typical night in the last two weeks?

1. none

2. a

3. two to three times

X 4. four to five times

5. very intense

11) Do you have difficulty picking up and using small objects, such as keys or pens?

1. without difficulty

2. little difficulty

3. moderate difficulty

X 4. Intense difficulty

5. very intense difficulty

A TYPICAL DAY, DURING THE LAST TWO

WEEKS, THE SYMPTOMS OF YOUR HAND OR WRIST

HAVE CAUSED HIM SOME DIFFICULTY IN

DO THE ACTIVITIES LISTED BELOW?

Please circle the number that best describes your ability to do each activity

ACTIVITY	DEGREE OF DIFFICULTY		
Writing	1 2 3 **X** 5		
Buttoning clothes	1 2 3 4 **X**		

Holding a book while reading	1 2 3 **X**	5
Holding the phone	1 2 3 **X**	5
Housework	1 2 3 **X**	5
Opening a bottle cap	1 2 3 4	**X**
Carrying grocery bags	1 2 3 4	**X**
Bathing and dressing	1 2 3 **X**	5

No difficulties 1

Little difficulty 2

Moderate difficulty 3

Intense difficulty 4

Can't do any work at all because of hand and wrist symptoms 5

Observer's opinion:

TABLE 5: Boston Questionnaire, clinical case 2, after 6 weeks of treatment

SELF-ASSESSMENT PROTOCOL - PROTOCOL

FROM BOSTON

Name: R. A.

Hand: (X) Right ( ) Left

Evaluation date: **2/6/2017**

THE FOLLOWING QUESTIONS REFER TO YOUR

SYMPTOMS IN A TYPICAL 24-HOUR PERIOD,

DURING THE LAST TWO WEEKS.

(Check one answer for each question)

1) How severe is the pain in your hand or wrist at night?

X 1. I have no pain in my hand or wrist at night

2. little pain

3. moderate pain

4. severe pain

5. very intense pain

2) How many times has pain in your hand or wrist woken you up during a typical night in the last two weeks?

X 1. None

2. a

3. two to three times

4. four to five times

5. more than five times

3) Do you usually have pain in your hand or wrist during the day?

X 1. I never have pain during the day

2. I have little pain during the day

3. I have moderate pain during the day

4. I have intense pain during the day

5. I have very intense pain during the day

4) How often do you get pain in your hand or wrist during the day?

X 1. never

2. once or twice a day

3. three to five times a day

4. more than five times a day

5. the pain is constant

5) How long, on average, do pain episodes last during the day?

X 1. I never have pain during the day

2. less than 10 minutes

3. from 10 to 60 minutes

4. more than 60 minutes

5. the pain is constant during the day

6) Do you have numbness (loss of feeling) in your hand?

X 1. no

2. I have little sleep

3. I have moderate numbness

4. I have intense numbness

5. I have very intense numbness

7) Do you have weakness in your hand or wrist?

X 1. no weakness

2. little weakness

3. moderate weakness

4. intense weakness

5. very intense weakness

8) Do you feel a tingling sensation in your hand?

X 1. No tingling

2. little tingling

3. moderate tingling

4. intense tingling

5. very intense tingling

9) How intense is the numbness (loss of feeling) or tingling at night?

X 1. I don't feel numb or tingly at night

2. little

3. moderate

4. intense

5. very intense

10) How often has numbness or tingling woken you up during a typical night in the last two weeks?

X 1. none

2. a

3. two to three times

4. four to five times

5. very intense

11) Do you have difficulty picking up and using small objects, such as keys or pens?

X 1. without difficulty

2. little difficulty

3. moderate difficulty

4. intense difficulty

5. very intense difficulty

A TYPICAL DAY, DURING THE LAST TWO

WEEKS, THE SYMPTOMS OF YOUR HAND OR WRIST

HAVE CAUSED HIM SOME DIFFICULTY IN

DO THE ACTIVITIES LISTED BELOW?

Please circle the number that best describes your ability to do each activity

ACTIVITY	DEGREE OF DIFFICULTY			
Writing	**X** 2	3	4	5
Buttoning clothes	**X** 2	3	4	5
Holding a book while reading	**X** 2	3	4	5
Holding the phone	**X** 2	3	4	5
Housework	**X** 2	3	4	5
Opening a bottle cap	**X** 2	3	4	5
Carrying grocery bags	**X** 2	3	4	5
Bathing and dressing	**X** 2	3	4	5

No difficulty 1

Little difficulty 2

Moderate difficulty 3

Intense difficulty 4

Can't do any work at all because of hand and wrist symptoms 5

Observer's opinion:

Case 3: A 63-year-old female office worker complained of severe pain in her right hand, with frequent numbness and numbness during the day and night. She was diagnosed with carpal tunnel syndrome around 15 months ago. She underwent various medical treatments, with little improvement. She began acupuncture treatments, to which she responded very favorably. He underwent twice-weekly treatments for six weeks, after which he showed a significant improvement in his symptoms, as can be seen in tables 6 and 7.

The patient verbalized that the symptoms she still sometimes reports are much less pronounced and do not interfere with her daily activities or her night's rest.

As far as grip strength is concerned, this was assessed before the treatments began and showed a marked decrease. Grip strength of the right hand: 8 kg.

After six weeks of treatment, grip strength of the right hand: 24 kg.

TABLE 6: Boston Questionnaire, clinical case 3, before the start of treatment

SELF-ASSESSMENT PROTOCOL - PROTOCOL

FROM BOSTON

Name: B. M.

Hand: (x) Right ( ) Left

Evaluation date: **23/4/2017**

THE FOLLOWING QUESTIONS REFER TO YOUR

SYMPTOMS IN A TYPICAL 24-HOUR PERIOD,

DURING THE LAST TWO WEEKS.

(Check one answer for each question)

1) How severe is the pain in your hand or wrist at night?

1. I have no pain in my hand or wrist at night

2. little pain

3. moderate pain

X 4. severe pain

5. very intense pain

2) How many times has pain in your hand or wrist woken you up during a typical night in the last two weeks?

1. none

2. a

3. two to three times

X 4. four to five times

5. more than five times

3) Do you usually have pain in your hand or wrist during the day?

1. I never have pain during the day

2. I have little pain during the day

3. I have moderate pain during the day

X 4. I have intense pain during the day

5. I have very intense pain during the day

4) How often do you get pain in your hand or wrist during the day?

1. never

2. once or twice a day

X 3. Three to five times a day

4. more than five times a day

5. the pain is constant

5) How long, on average, do pain episodes last during the day?

1. I never have pain during the day

2. less than 10 minutes

X 3. 10 to 60 minutes

4. more than 60 minutes

5. the pain is constant during the day

6) Do you have numbness (loss of feeling) in your hand?

1. no

2. I have little sleep

3. I have moderate numbness

4. I have intense numbness

X 5. I have very intense numbness

7) Do you have weakness in your hand or wrist?

1. no weakness

2. little weakness

3. moderate weakness

4. intense weakness

X 5. very intense weakness

8) Do you feel a tingling sensation in your hand?

1. no tingling

2. little tingling

3. moderate tingling

X 4. Intense tingling

5. very intense tingling

9) How intense is the numbness (loss of feeling) or tingling at night?

1. I don't feel numb or tingly at night

2. little

3. moderate

4. intense

X 5. very intense

10) How often has numbness or tingling woken you up during a typical night in the last two weeks?

1. none

2. a

3. two to three times

X 4. four to five times

5. very intense

11) Do you have difficulty picking up and using small objects, such as keys or pens?

1. without difficulty

2. little difficulty

3. moderate difficulty

X 4. Intense difficulty

5. very intense difficulty

A TYPICAL DAY, DURING THE LAST TWO

WEEKS, THE SYMPTOMS OF YOUR HAND OR WRIST

HAVE CAUSED HIM SOME DIFFICULTY IN

DO THE ACTIVITIES LISTED BELOW?

Please circle the number that best describes your ability to do each activity

ACTIVITY   **DEGREE OF**

Writing	**DIFFICULTY**				
	1 2	3	**X**		5
Buttoning clothes	1 2	3	**X**		5
Holding a book while reading	1 2	3	**X**		5
Holding the phone	1 2	3	**X**		5
Housework	1 2	3	**X**		5
Opening a bottle cap	1 2	3	4	**X**	
Carrying grocery bags	1 2	3	4	**X**	
Bathing and dressing	1 2	3	**X**		5

No difficulties 1

Little difficulty 2

Moderate difficulty 3

Intense difficulty 4

Can't do any work at all because of hand and wrist symptoms 5

Observer's opinion: ____

____

TABLE 7: Boston questionnaire clinical case 3, after 6 weeks of treatment

SELF-ASSESSMENT PROTOCOL - PROTOCOL

FROM BOSTON

Name: B. M.

Hand: (x) Right ( ) Left D

evaluation minutes: **23/4/2017**

THE FOLLOWING QUESTIONS REFER TO YOUR

SYMPTOMS IN A TYPICAL 24-HOUR PERIOD,

DURING THE LAST TWO WEEKS.

(Check one answer for each question)

1) How severe is the pain in your hand or wrist at night?

1. I have no pain in my hand or wrist at night

X 2. Little pain

3. moderate pain

4. severe pain

5. very intense pain

2) How many times has pain in your hand or wrist woken you up during a typical night in the last two weeks?

1. none

X 2. a

3. two to three times

4. four to five times

5. more than five times

3) Do you usually have pain in your hand or wrist during the day?

X 1. I never have pain during the day

2. I have little pain during the day

3. I have moderate pain during the day

4. I have intense pain during the day

5. I have very intense pain during the day

4) How often do you get pain in your hand or wrist during the day?

X 1. never

2. once or twice a day

3. three to five times a day

4. more than five times a day

5. the pain is constant

5) How long, on average, do pain episodes last during the day?

X 1. I never have pain during the day

2. less than 10 minutes

3. from 10 to 60 minutes

4. more than 60 minutes

5. the pain is constant during the day

6) Do you have numbness (loss of feeling) in your hand?

1. no

X 2. I have little sleep

3. I have moderate numbness

4. I have intense numbness

5. I have very intense numbness

7) Do you have weakness in your hand or wrist?

1. no weakness

X 2. Little weakness

3. moderate weakness

4. intense weakness

5. very intense weakness

8) Do you feel a tingling sensation in your hand?

X 1. No tingling

2. little tingling

3. moderate tingling

4. intense tingling

Observer's opinion:

9) How intense is the numbness (loss of feeling) or tingling at night?

1. I don't feel numb or tingly at night

X 2. little

3. moderate

4. intense

5. very intense

10) How often has numbness or tingling woken you up during a typical night in the last two weeks?

X 1. None

2. a

3. two to three times

4. four to five times

5. very intense

11) Do you have difficulty picking up and using small objects, such as keys or pens? 1. no difficulty

X 2. little difficulty

3. moderate difficulty

4. intense difficulty

5. very intense difficulty

A TYPICAL DAY, DURING THE LAST TWO

WEEKS, THE SYMPTOMS OF YOUR HAND OR WRIST

HAVE CAUSED HIM SOME DIFFICULTY IN

DO THE ACTIVITIES LISTED BELOW?

Please circle the number that best describes your ability to do each activity

ACTIVITY   **GRADE OF DIFFICULTY**

Activity					
Writing	X	2	3	4	5
Buttoning clothes	X	2	3	4	5
Holding a book while reading	X	2	3	4	5
Holding the phone	X	2	3	4	5
Housework	1	X	3	4	5
Opening a bottle cap	1	X	3	4	5
Carrying grocery bags	1	X	3	4	5
Bathing and dressing	X	2	3	4	5

No difficulties 1

Little difficulty 2

Moderate difficulty 3

Intense difficulty 4

She can't do any work because of the symptoms of her hands and wrists 5

5. very intense tingling

Case 4: A 33-year-old woman, employed in an accounting office, presented with intense pain in her right hand, accompanied by tingling and numbness, symptoms which severely restricted her work activity and led to frequent sick leave. She also had great difficulty doing household chores. About 12 months ago, she was diagnosed with carpal tunnel syndrome. She was put on analgesic medication for several periods, without any significant improvement. He was also given corticosteroids and used them night and day, quite frequently.

She started acupuncture treatments and saw significant improvements after the first treatment. She underwent twice-weekly treatments for six weeks and there was a marked reduction in symptoms, as can be seen in tables 8 and 9. According to the patient, the pain disappeared completely, with only some numbness remaining after periods of increased work effort. She no longer needed to take analgesic medication or use an immobilizing splint.

With regard to the grip strength of her right hand, before starting treatment, she had very low strength, which resulted in a high degree of disability. Right hand grip strength before treatment: 6 kg. After 6 weeks of acupuncture treatment, the grip strength of the right hand improved significantly, which, together with the remission of symptoms, greatly increased the patient's quality of life.

Right hand grip strength after 6 weeks of treatment: 26 kg.

TABLE 8: Boston Questionnaire, clinical case 4, before the start of treatment

SELF-ASSESSMENT PROTOCOL - PROTOCOL

FROM BOSTON

Name: S. S.

Hand: (x) Right ( ) Left

Date of evaluation: **16/5/2017**

THE FOLLOWING QUESTIONS REFER TO YOUR

SYMPTOMS IN A TYPICAL 24-HOUR PERIOD,

DURING THE LAST TWO WEEKS.

(Check one answer for each question)

1) How severe is the pain in your hand or wrist at night?

1. I have no pain in my hand or wrist at night

2. little pain

3. moderate pain

4. severe pain

X 5. Very intense pain

2) How many times has pain in your hand or wrist woken you up during a typical night in the last two weeks?

1. none

2. a

3. two to three times

4. four to five times

X 5. more than five times

3) Do you usually have pain in your hand or wrist during the day?

1. I never have pain during the day

2. I have little pain during the day

3. I have moderate pain during the day

4. I have intense pain during the day

X 5. I have very intense pain during the day

4) How often do you get pain in your hand or wrist during the day?

1. never

2. once or twice a day

3. three to five times a day

4. more than five times a day

X 5. pain is constant

5) How long, on average, do pain episodes last during the day?

1. I never have pain during the day

2. less than 10 minutes

3. from 10 to 60 minutes

4. more than 60 minutes

X 5. the pain is constant during the day

6) Do you have numbness (loss of feeling) in your hand?

1. no

2. I have little sleep

3. I have moderate numbness

4. I have intense numbness

X 5. I have very intense numbness

7) Do you have weakness in your hand or wrist?

1. no weakness

2. little weakness

3. moderate weakness

4. intense weakness

X 5. very intense weakness

8) Do you feel a tingling sensation in your hand?

1. no tingling

2. little tingling

3. moderate tingling

4. intense tingling

X 5. Very intense tingling

9) How intense is the numbness (loss of feeling) or tingling at night?

1. I don't feel numb or tingly at night

2. little

3. moderate

4. intense

X 5. very intense

10) How often has numbness or tingling woken you up during a typical night in the last two weeks?

1. none

2. a

3. two to three times

4. four to five times

X 5. very intense

11) Do you have difficulty picking up and using small objects, such as keys or pens?

1. without difficulty

2. little difficulty

3. moderate difficulty

4. intense difficulty

X 5. very intense difficulty ON A TYPICAL DAY, DURING THE LAST TWO

WEEKS, THE SYMPTOMS OF YOUR HAND OR WRIST

HAVE CAUSED HIM SOME DIFFICULTY IN

DO THE ACTIVITIES LISTED BELOW?

Please circle the number that best describes your ability to do each activity

ACTIVITY	DEGREE OF DIFFICULTY			
Writing	1 2	3	**X**	5
Buttoning clothes	1 2	3	**X**	5
Holding a book while reading	1 2	3	4	**X**
Holding the phone	1 2	3	**X**	5
Housework	1 2	3	**X**	5
Opening a bottle cap	1 2	3	4	**X**
Carrying grocery bags	1 2	3	4	**X**
Bathing and dressing	1 2	3	**X**	5

No difficulties 1

Little difficulty 2

Moderate difficulty 3

Intense difficulty 4

She can't do any work at all because of the symptoms in her hands and wrists 5

Observer's opinion: ____

TABLE 9: Boston Questionnaire, clinical case 4, after 6 weeks of treatment

SELF-ASSESSMENT PROTOCOL - PROTOCOL

FROM BOSTON

Name: S. S.

Hand: (x) Right ( ) Left

Evaluation date: **9/6/2017**

THE FOLLOWING QUESTIONS REFER TO YOUR

SYMPTOMS IN A TYPICAL 24-HOUR PERIOD,

DURING THE LAST TWO WEEKS.

(Check one answer for each question)

1) How severe is the pain in your hand or wrist at night?

X1. I have no pain in my hand or wrist at night

2. little pain

3. moderate pain

4. severe pain

5. very intense pain

2) How many times has pain in your hand or wrist woken you up during a typical night in the last two weeks?

X 1. none

2. a

3. two to three times

4. four to five times

5. more than five times

3) Do you usually have pain in your hand or wrist during the day?

X 1. I never have pain during the day

2. I have little pain during the day

3. I have moderate pain during the day

4. I have intense pain during the day

5. I have very intense pain during the day

4) How often do you get pain in your hand or wrist during the day?

X 1. never

2. once or twice a day

3. three to five times a day

4. more than five times a day

5. the pain is constant

5) How long, on average, do pain episodes last during the day?

X 1. I never have pain during the day

2. less than 10 minutes

3. from 10 to 60 minutes

4. more than 60 minutes

5. the pain is constant during the day

6) Do you have numbness (loss of feeling) in your hand?

1. no

X 2. I have little sleep

3. I have moderate numbness

4. I have intense numbness

5. I have very intense numbness

7) Do you have weakness in your hand or wrist?

1. no weakness

X 2. Little weakness

3. moderate weakness

4. intense weakness

5. very intense weakness

8) Do you feel a tingling sensation in your hand?

X 1. No tingling

2. little tingling

3. moderate tingling

4. intense tingling

5. very intense tingling

9) How intense is the numbness (loss of sensation) or tingling at night?

X 1. I don't feel numb or tingly at night

2. little

3. moderate

4. intense

5. very intense

10) How often has numbness or tingling woken you up during a typical night in the last two weeks?

X 1. none

2. a

3. two to three times

4. four to five times

5. very intense

11) Do you have difficulty picking up and using small objects, such as keys or pens? 1. no difficulty

X 2. little difficulty

3. moderate difficulty

4. intense difficulty

5. very intense difficulty

A TYPICAL DAY, DURING THE LAST TWO

WEEKS, THE SYMPTOMS OF YOUR HAND OR WRIST

HAVE CAUSED HIM SOME DIFFICULTY IN

DO THE ACTIVITIES LISTED BELOW?

Please circle the number that best describes your ability to do each activity

ACTIVITY	DEGREE OF DIFFICULTY				
Writing	**X**	2	3	4	5
Buttoning clothes	1	**X**	3	4	5
Holding a book while reading	**X**	2	3	4	5
Holding the phone	**X**	2	3	4	5
Housework	1	**X**	3	4	5
Opening a bottle cap	1	**X**	3	4	5
Carrying grocery bags	1	**X**	3	4	5
Bathing and dressing	**X**	2	3	4	5

No difficulties 1

Little difficulty 2

Moderate difficulty 3

Intense difficulty 4

Can't do any work at all because of hand and wrist symptoms 5

Observer's opinion: ____

The results obtained in the treatment of the patients presented above reinforce the premise that acupuncture can be an effective alternative for controlling the symptoms of carpal tunnel syndrome. The four patients presented in the clinical cases were contacted by telephone four weeks after the last treatment to check whether the improvements had been maintained, and the patients confirmed that the results had remained unchanged. Acupuncture seems to be an effective and long-lasting alternative for reducing symptoms in carpal tunnel syndrome.

In this way, and based on the small sample size of this study, motivated by the time limit, we consider it of great importance to develop studies in this area, as a way of validating and generalizing the results obtained.

These results seem to be in line with the literature. However, the scientific validity of some of the studies found, and referred to throughout the text, is still questioned by the researchers themselves, due to the difficulty in separating the effect of acupuncture per se from the placebo effect.

4. Discussion and Conclusions

The carpal canal is the narrowest at the level of the hook of the hamate. In turn, the median nerve is the most superficial structure within it and is connected to other surrounding structures, namely the tendons that innervate the fingers, among others (Rotman & Donovan, 2002). The narrowing of this canal, caused by numerous possible causes mentioned above, causes compression in these structures, which in turn produces a set of symptoms known as carpal tunnel syndrome.

Carpal canal syndrome is one of the most prevalent peripheral neuropathies (Khosrawi et al, 2012) whose symptoms significantly interfere with the performance of activities of daily living, causing a reduction in the quality of life of affected individuals.

The figures found in terms of incidence and prevalence of this pathology demonstrate its importance to the medical community. Chammas and colleagues (2014) report that the prevalence of CHS, estimated for the general population, varies between 4% and 5% and particularly affects individuals between the ages of 40 and 60. The same authors point out that in 2008, 127,269 individuals aged 20 or over underwent surgical intervention to treat CCS in metropolitan France, giving an incidence of 2.7/1000 (Women: 3.6/1000; Men: 1.7/1000). They also point out that there are two peaks of frequency, the first and highest being between the ages of 49 and 59, in which the vast majority (75%) are women; and the second peak is between the ages of 75 and 84, in which women account for 64%.

Yunoki et al. (2017) also report that 1 to 4% of the general population suffers from this condition, with 1 to 2 individuals out of every 5 suffering from symptoms of pain, tingling and numbness in the upper extremities being diagnosed with carpal tunnel syndrome. The annual incidence of this condition is 276/100,000 inhabitants. The same authors point out that it is more common in women, with a two-thirds to one-third ratio between women and men. Mondelli and

collaborators (2002) state that the development of this pathology is also related to age. Although it is seen in all age groups, it has a higher incidence in the 40-60 age group. The same authors point out that only 10% occur before the age of 30. In the same vein, Bugajska et al. (2007) add that the incidence also increases with the number of years worked. It should be noted that the fact that the pathology is more common in the elderly means that there is a more marked decrease in the mobility and independence of the elderly in carrying out activities of daily living.

Existing therapeutic responses do not provide satisfactory and definitive results, and there is often a recurrence of symptoms and associated limitations. There is therefore an urgent need to find new forms of treatment, both pharmacological and non-pharmacological, which, combined with the development of new health education strategies, will guarantee that individuals can better meet their needs.

It is in this sense that TCM presents itself as a therapeutic approach to be considered in the reduction of pain associated with musculoskeletal disorders. As far as carpal tunnel syndrome is concerned, there are already a considerable number of studies that seem to indicate the effectiveness of acupuncture in controlling its symptoms. However, taking into account that this condition is still quite recent, having been described for the first time by Brain et al. in 1947, we consider it extremely important to carry out more studies in this area.

The bibliographic research found is generally in line with the results observed in the patients presented in this study. We would like to highlight the study carried out by Khosrawi et al. in 2012, which found that 71.9% of patients undergoing acupuncture treatment were female, with an average age of 41.7 years, ranging from 25 to 65 years old. In their conclusions on the effectiveness of acupuncture, the authors state that it can generally improve symptoms related to CFS. However, the authors point out that, due to the small sample size and the short period of time in which the study took place, it has some limitations in terms of its scientific validity. Kumnerddee and Kaewtong (2010) also carried out a study aimed at comparing the effectiveness of acupuncture with the use of a night splint in controlling the symptoms of CCS and concluded that electroacupuncture was just as effective as the use of the splint in controlling symptoms in general and improving function. However, acupuncture was more effective in controlling pain.

In 2010, Ashworth carried out a systematic review of the literature, the aim of which was to assess the effectiveness of various therapeutic approaches, both pharmacological and non-pharmacological, in controlling the symptoms of CFS. This study compared the various alternatives presented and concluded that, in relation to both acupuncture and massage therapy, no clinically important results were found regarding the effect of these therapeutic approaches in the treatment of CCS. Despite these discouraging results, Khosrawi et al. in 2012 highlighted the fact that the US National Institute of Health (NIH), which is part of the US Department of Health and Human Services and is responsible for US medical research, has confirmed that acupuncture is a proven treatment for the control of mild to moderate symptoms of CFS.

These results are supported by Lundeberg (1999) cited by Freedman (2017) who justifies the effect of acupuncture in reducing the symptoms associated with CCS, explaining that it offers relief of local symptoms, possibly by reducing edema, as a result of the release of neuropeptides by the sensory nerves.

Wang and colleagues (2008) consulted multiple medical databases in order to prove the effect of acupuncture on pain control and concluded that acupuncture, as well as other forms of stimulation, were effective in controlling pain in the short term in various pathologies, including CCS.

Sim and colleagues (2011) also carried out a systematic review of the literature, using electronic databases and whose methodological quality was assessed by Cochrane, with the aim of testing the effectiveness of acupuncture in controlling the symptoms of CFS. The authors concluded that the existing scientific evidence is not strong enough to suggest that acupuncture is an effective treatment for CCS, although there is some evidence of its usefulness.

However, the results obtained in the 4 clinical cases unequivocally corroborate the evidence found in a significant number of the bibliographies consulted. By analyzing the clinical cases that formed the basis of this study, we can see that, with regard to the patient in case 1, and the intensity of her symptoms, she had severe pain, the intensity of which woke her up 2-3 times a night. During the day, the pain was very intense and constant. In addition to the pain, the patient also reported very intense numbness and weakness, and intense tingling. At night, the tingling was very intense and she woke up 2-3 times a night as a result. She also had intense difficulty picking up and using small objects, such as keys or pens. She was completely unable to carry out activities of daily living, as shown in Table 2.

After 4 weeks of treatment, the *grip strength* quadrupled in both hands, going from 10 kg to 40 kg in the right hand and from 8 kg to 35 kg in the left hand. As can be seen in table 3, the symptoms presented completely regressed and there were no symptoms or limitations in carrying out daily activities.

Turning to case 2, the patient reported intense symptoms, with serious implications for her quality of life, particularly in terms of resting at night, due to the number of times she woke up during the night as a result of her symptoms. She had intense difficulty performing simple daily activities, as shown in Table 4. After the treatments carried out, all the symptoms completely regressed, as did the difficulty in carrying out daily activities (chart 5). Handgrip strength tripled from 8 kg before treatment to 25 kg after treatment.

With regard to case 3, we can see from table 6 that the patient had severe pain, with serious implications for her rest at night, which continued throughout the day, occurring 3 to 5 times a day, with episodes lasting between 10 and 60 minutes. She also had very intense numbness and weakness and intense tingling. With regard to daily activities, she had intense difficulty in carrying them out, with a total inability to open jar lids or carry supermarket bags. After the treatments, as shown in table 7, we can see that her symptoms improved significantly, with only very slight pain or numbness and sporadic onset. As for the difficulty in carrying out daily activities, there was a very significant improvement.

doing housework, opening jar lids or carrying supermarket bags.

The pressing force tripled from 8 kg to 24 kg.

The patient in case 4 had very intense symptoms, as can be seen in table 8. In addition to these results, she also had very intense difficulty in carrying out the various daily activities listed in the Boston questionnaire, and a total inability to open jar lids or carry supermarket bags. After the treatments, and according to the information in Table 9, we found that the symptoms improved very significantly, with a complete absence of pain. The weakness, numbness and tingling were very slight and sporadic. With regard to the difficulties reported in carrying out daily activities, these have reduced significantly, with only slight difficulty in buttoning clothes, doing some housework, opening jar lids and carrying supermarket bags.

Pressing force also quadrupled, from 6 kg before treatment to 26 kg after treatment.

Based on the results obtained in this pilot study and its importance in terms of improving the quality of life of users, we consider it very pertinent to repeat this study, in a sample whose size is representative of the population with carpal tunnel syndrome, in order to allow the extrapolation of the results to the general population, a fact that has motivated us to present a proposal for a research protocol, which is shown in Annex 2.

Based on the adequate size of the suggested sample and by extrapolating the results found in the clinical cases presented to this sample, we believe we can clearly demonstrate, through the possible findings, the effect of acupuncture in controlling the symptoms of CCS.

From the literature consulted, we can see that acupuncture is a valid alternative for controlling the symptoms of this pathology. Citing Yang et al. (2009), we can say that short-term acupuncture treatment is as effective as low-dose prednisolone, also in the short term, for controlling the symptoms of mild to moderate CCS. Thus, the authors emphasize that for those who have intolerance or contraindication to the use of oral steroids or for those who do not opt for early surgery, acupuncture treatment offers an alternative choice.

Khosrawi and colleagues (2012) also point out that the findings of their study indicated that acupuncture can improve the overall subjective symptoms of carpal tunnel syndrome and can be adopted in comprehensive care programs for these patients.

In this sense, we also cite Yang et al. (2010), whose study aimed to evaluate the long-term effect of acupuncture on patients with CCS, who found that the experimental group showed a more significant improvement in symptomatology, motor function and sensitivity of the affected limb, when compared to the group that took oral steroids one year after the end of treatment. These authors concluded that short-term acupuncture treatment can result in long-term improvement in mild to moderate idiopathic CFS. They point out that acupuncture treatment can be considered as an alternative therapy to other conservative treatments for patients who do not opt for early surgical decompression.

Finally, we present the results of a clinical case carried out by Norman in 2010, whose results are similar to those observed in this study. The author reports the case of a 62-year-old woman with pain and weakness in both hands who, after the first acupuncture session, reported a 70% reduction in pain and normal grip strength. The author points out that the reduction in pain remained at 70% until a further assessment after 6 months. The author concludes that acupuncture can quickly open energy blockages and release myofascial spasms, which contribute to carpal tunnel syndrome symptoms.

These results allow us to realize the long road we still have to travel, *but the path is made by walking,* as Fernando Pessoa would say, and I believe we will reach our destination, which is to validate the effectiveness of acupuncture in treating this pathology.

5. BIBLIOGRAPHICAL REFERENCES

Aroori, S. & Spence, R. (2008). Carpal Tunnel Syndrome. *Ulster Med J.*; 77 (1) 6-17.

Ashworth, N. (2009). Carpal Tunnel Syndrome. *Clinical Evidence.* 03:1114.

Berman, B.M., Lao, L., Langerberg, P.,Lee, W.L., Gilpin, A.M., Hochberg, M.C. (2004) Effectiveness of acupuncture as adjunctive therapy in osteoarthritis of the knee:a randomized controlled trial. *Ann Intern Med*; 21:902-20.

Bland, J. (2007). Steroid injection and surgical decompression in Carpal Tunnel Syndrome. *Muscle Nerve*; 36: 167-171.

Branco, K. & Naeser, M. (1999*).* Carpal tunnel syndrome: clinical outcome after low-level laser acupuncture, microamperes transcutaneous electrical nerve stimulation, and other alternative therapies-an open protocol study. *The journal of alternative and complementary medicine.* 5 (1): 5-26.

Bugajska, J.; Jedryka-Góral, A.; Sudol-Szopinska, I. (2007). Carpal Tunnel Syndrome in occupational Medicine Practice. *International Journal of Occupational Safety and Ergonomics (JOSE).* 13 (1): 29-38.

Campos, C.; Manzano, G.; Andrade, L. et al. (2003). Translation and validation of the questionnaire for assessing symptom severity and functional status in carpal tunnel syndrome. *Arq. Neuropsiquiatr.* 61(1):51-55.

Chammas M, Boretto J, Burmann LM, Ramos RM, dos Santos Neto FC, Silva JB. (2014). Carpal tunnel syndrome - Part I (anatomy, physiology, etiology and diagnosis). *Rev Bras Ortop.* 49(5):429-36.

Chung, V., Robin, S.T., Liu, S., Marc, K.C.,et al (2016) Electroacupuncture and splinting versus splinting alone to treat carpal tunnel syndrome: a randomized controlled trial. *CMAJ,* September 6, 188 (6).

De-feng, CAI (2010). Relaxing for the Treatment of Carpal Tunnel Syndrome. *Journal of traditional Chinese Medicine.* March. 3 (1).

Ernst, E. (2006). Acupuncture - a critical anlysis. *Journal of Internal Medicine,* 259, 125137.

Fortin, M.F. (2009). *Fundamentals and stages of the research process.* Lusodidacta. Loures, 595 p.

Freedman, J. (2017). *Acupuncture for carpal tunnel syndrome.* Download from: http409 p.://aim.bmj.com/ on June 4, 2017 - Published by group.bmj.com

Greten, H. (2007). *Understanding Chinese Pharmacology. Scientific Chinese Medicine.* Heidelberg: Heidelberg School Editions. Unrevised course version 2016.

Greten, H. (2011). *Understanding TCM-Scientific Chinese Medicine.* Course Version (5ed). Heidelberg: Heidelberg School Editions.

Greten, H. (2007). *Understanding TCM - The Fundamentals of Chinese Medicine, Part I.* Heidelberg: Heidelberg Shool Editions, 6th rev. ed. 2013.

Greten, H. (2015). *Understanding TCM - The Fundamentals of Chinese Medicine, Part II.* Heidelberg: Heidelberg School Editions.

Greten, H. (2016). *Clinical Subjects - Scientific Chinese Medicine.* Heidelberg: Heidelberg School Editions.

Gurcay, A.G.; Karaahmet, O.Z.; Gurcan, O.; et al (2016). Comparison of short-term clinical and electrophysiological outcomes of Local Steroid Injection and Surgical Decompression in the Treatment of Carpal Tunnel Syndrome. *Turk Neurosurg.* 27(3): 447-452; DOI: 10.5137/1019-5149.JTN.15936-15.0

Hadianfard, M.; Bazrafshan, E.; Momeninejad, H.; Jahani, N. (2015). Efficacies of Acupuncture and Anti-inflammatory Treatment for Carpal Tunnel Syndrome. *Journal of acupuncture and Meridian Studies*; 8(5): 229-235.

Hempen, C.; Chow, V. (2006). *Pocket Atlas of Acupuncture.* Thieme. New York. 304 p.

Ho Cy, Lin HC, Lee YC et al (2014). Clinical effectiveness of acupuncture for carpal tunnel syndrome. *Am J Chin Med.*; 42(2):303-14. doi: 10.1142/S0192415X14500207.

Hong, J.; Lee, S.; Han, S.; Son, B. et al (2006). Anatomy of neurovascular structures around the carpal tunnel during dynamic wrist motion for endoscopic carpal tunnel release. *Neurosurgery.* Feb; 58(1 Suppl.) ONS 127-33.

Huisstede, B.M.; Van den Brink, J.; Randsdorp, M.S.; et al (2017). Effetiveness of Surgical and Postsurgical Interventions for Carpal Tunnel Syndrome - A systematic Review. *Arch. Phys. Med. Rehabil.* May: 31. Doi: 10.1016/j.apmr.201704.024.

Kanaan, N. & Sawaya, R. (2001). Carpal Tunnel Syndrome: modern diagnostic and management techniques. *British Journal of General Practice*; 51, 311-314.

Kim, J.K.; Koh, Y.; Kim, J.O.; et al (2016). Changes in Clinical Symptoms, Functions, and the Median Nerve Cross-sectional Area at the Carpal Tunnel Inlet after Open Carpal Tunnel Release. *Clinics in Orthopedic Surgery.* 8; 298-302.

Khosrawi, S.; Moghtaderi, A.; Haghighat, s. (2012). Acupuncture in treatment of carpal tunnel syndrome: A randomized controlled trial study. *Journal of Research in Medical Sciences.* Jan; 17(1): 1-7.

Kubiena, G.; Sommer, B. (2004). *Practice Handbook of acupuncture.* Churchill Livingstone. UK. 3rd ed.

Kumar S, Beaton K, Hughes T. (2013). The effectiveness of massage therapy for the treatment of nonspecific low back pain: a systematic review of systematic reviews. *Int J General Med.* 6:733.

Kumnerddee, W.; Kaewtong, A. (2010). Efficacy of acupuncture versus night splinting for carpal tunnel syndrome: a randomized clinical trial. *J Med Assoc Thai.* Dec; 93(12): 1463-9.

Leigh, J.P., Miller T.R. (1998). Job-related diseases and occupations within a large workers' compensation data set. *Am J Ind Med*, 33: 197-211.

Lewis, M. & Johnson, M. (2006). *The clinical effectiveness of therapeutic massage for musculoskeletal pain: a systematic review. Database of Abstracts of Reviews of Effects* (DARE): Quality-assessed Reviews [Internet].

https://www.ncbi.nlm.nih.gov/pubmedhealth/PMH0023286/

Meirelles, L.; Santos, J.; santos, L.; Branco, M. et al. (2006). Evaluation of the Boston questionnaire applied in the late postoperative period of carpal tunnel syndrome operated by the Paine retinaculotome technique via the palmar approach. *Acta Ortop Bras.* 14 (3): 126132.

Mondelli M., Giannini F., Giachi M. (2002) Carpal tunnel syndrome incidence in a general population. *Neurology*, 58: 289-294.

Naslund, J., Naslund, U., & Odenbring, S. (2002). Sensory Stimulation (acupuncture) for the Treatment of Idiopathic Anterior Knee Pain. *Journal Rehabilitation of Medicine*, 34, 231-238.

NIH Consensus Conference (1998). Acupuncture. JAMA. Nov 4;280(17):1518-24.

Nobuta, S.; sato, K.; Nakagawa, T.; Hatori, M.; Itoi, E. (2017). Effects of Wrist Splinting for Carpal Tunnel Syndrome and Motor Nerve Conduction Measurements. *Upsala Journal of Medical Sciences.* 113 (2): 181-192.

Nghi, N.; Dzung, T.; Recours-Nguyen, C. (2004). *Art and Practice of Acupuncture and Moxibustion.* Roca. São Paulo, 644 p.

Norman, Z. (2010). Acupuncture Treatment for Carpal Tunnel Syndrome. *Medical Acupuncture.* December 2010, Vol. 22, No. 4: 273-276

Porkert, M. (1983). *The Essentials of Chinese Diagnostics* (Vol. 3). Zurich, Switzerland: Acta Medicinae Sinensis Chinese Medicine Publications LTD.

Porkert, M. (2001). *Chinese Medical Diagnostics a ComprehensiveTextbook.*

Shcafflertrasse, Dinkelscherben, Germany: European Edition.

Porkert, M., & Hempen, C.H. (1995). *Classical Acupuncture - The Standard Textbook.* Schafflerstrasse, Dinkelscherben, Germany: Phainon Editions & Media GmbH Acta Medicinae sinensis.

Prime, M.S., Palmer, J., Khan, W.S., Goddard, N.J. (2010). Is there light at the end of the tunnel? Controversies in the diagnosis and management of carpal tunnel syndrome. *HAND*, 5: 354-360.

Rotman, M.; Donovan, J. (2002). Practical anatomy of the carpal tunnel. *Hand Clin.* May; 18(2): 219-30.

Sim, H.; Shin, B.; Lee, M.; Ernst, E. (2011). Acupuncture for carpal tunnel syndrome: a systemic review of randomized controlled trials. *Pain.* Mar; 12(3):307-14. doi: 10.1016/j.jpain.2010.08.006.

Sousa, C.; Moreira, L.; Coimbra, D.; Machado, J.; Greten, H. (2015). Immediate effects of Tuina techniques on working-related musculosketal disorder of professional orchestra musicians. *Journal of Integrative Medicine.* July, vol.13, N°4.

Tsao, J. (2007). Effectiveness of Massage Therapy for Chronic, Non-malignant Pain: A Review. *Evid Based Complement Alternat Med.* Jun; 4(2): 165-179.

Vieira, A. (2003). Management of Carpal Tunnel Syndrome. *American Family Physician.* Volume 68, Number 2, July 15.

Walker, W.C., Metzler, M., Cifu, D.X., Swartz, Z. (2000) Neutral wrist splinting in carpal tunnel syndrome; a comparison of night-only versus full-time wear instructions. *Arch Phys Med Rehabil.* 81: 424-429.

Wang, S.; Kain, Z.; White, P. (2008). Acupuncture Analgesia II: Clinical Considerations. *Anesthesia & Analgesia.* Feb:106 (2): 611-621.

Wipperman, J.; Goerl, K. (2016). Carpal Tunnel Syndrome: Diagnosis and management. *Am Fam Physician.* Dec; 15; 94(12): 993-999.

Yang, C.P.; Hsieh, C.L.; Wang, N.H. et al (2009). Acupuncture in patients with carpal tunnel syndrome: a randomized controlled trial. *Clin. J. Pain* 25:327-333. PubMed: 19590482.

yang, c.p.; wang, n.h.; li, t.c. et al (2010). A randomized clinical trial of acupuncture versus oral steroids for carpal tunnel syndrome: a long-term follow-up. *Journal of*

Pain. Feb;12(2):272-9. doi: 10.1016/j.jpain.2010.09.001.

Yang, M.; Feng, Y.; Pei, H.; Deng, S. et al. (2014). *Effectiveness of Chinese massage therapy (Tui Na) for chronic low back pain: study protocol for a randomized controlled trial.* Trials 2014, 15:418. http://www.trialsjoumal.eom/content/15/1/418

Yunoki, M.; Kanda, T.; Suzuki, K.; Hirashita, K.; et al (2017). Importance of Recognizing Carpal Tunnel Syndrome for Neurosurgeons: a Review. *Neurol Med Chir* (Tokyo) April, 57, 172-183.

6. ANNEXES

ANNEX 1 : Boston Self-Assessment Questionnaire

ANNEX 1

SELF-ASSESSMENT PROTOCOL -

BOSTON PROTOCOL

Name: . ...

RGHSP MAo:.( ) Right ( ) Left

Evaluation Date ... Date of C| rurg| a

THE FOLLOWING QUESTIONS REFER TO YOUR SYMPTOMS IN A TYPICAL 24-HOUR PERIOD OVER THE LAST TWO WEEKS.

(Choose one answer for each question)

1) How does the pain in your hand or wrist get worse at night?

1-   I don't get pain in my hand or wrist at night

2-   little pain

3· mode pain

4-   intense pain

5-   very intense pain

2) How many times has pain in your hand or wrist woken you up during a typical night in the last two weeks?

1-   none

2-one

3-   two to three times

4-   four to five times

5-   more than five times

3) Do you usually have pain in your hand or wrist during the day?

1-   I never have pain during the day

2-   i have little pain during the day 3- i have moderate pain during the day

4-   I have intense pain during the day

5-   I have very intense pain during the day

4) How often do you get pain in your hand or wrist during the day?

1-never

2-   once or twice a day

3-   three to five times a day

4-   more than five times a day

5-   the pain is constant

5) How long, on average, do da episodes last during the day?

1-   I never have da during o day

2- less than 10 minutes

3-   from 10 to 60 minutes

4-   more than 60 minutes

5-   the pain is constant throughout the day

6) Do you have numbness (loss of feeling) in your hand?

1-   no

2-   I'm not very big

3-   I have moderate adcrmedmento

4-   I have intense adamancy

5-   I have intense bush love

7) Do you have Iraqueza in your hand or wrist?

1-without anger

2-   little weakness

3-   moderate weakness

4-   intense weakness

5-   very intense weakness

8) You have a feeling of numbness in your hand'

1-   no lanvgamento

2-   little tingling

3-   moderate tingling

4-   intense tingling

5-   very intense tingling

9) How intense is the numbness (loss of sensation) or tingling at night?

1-   - i don't fall asleep or get dizzy at night

2-   little

3- moderate

4- intense

5- very intense

10) How often has Oadormedmento or oform | да- mento woken you up during a typical night in the last two weeks'

1-none

2- a

3- two to three times

4- four to five times

5- very intense

11) Do you have difficulty picking up and using small objects such as keys or pens?

1- without difficulty

2- little officiousness

3- moderate difficulty

4- intense difficulty

5- very intense difficulty

ONE TYPICAL DAY DURING THE LAST TWO WEEKS, HAVE THE SYMPTOMS IN YOUR HAND OR FIST CAUSED YOU ANY DIFFICULTY IN DOING THE ACTIVITIES USED BELOW?

Pa fava circle o number that describes your ability to make alidade

ATIVI DAOE	DEGREE OF QUALIFICATION			
Esaever	1	2	3	4 5
Buttoning clothes	1	2	3	4 5
Holding an Irvro while reading	1	2	3	4 5
Hold o phone	1	2	3	4 5
Housework	1	2	3	4 5
Opening a glass lid	1	2	3	-1 5
Canegarsacos Ce Sipermercaccs	1	2	3	4 5
Shower and get dressed	1	2	3	4 5

No difficulties	1
Little difficulty	...2
Moderate difficulty	3
Intense difficulty	.4

There's no way you'll be able to make

61

a mistake,

for hand and wrist symptoms ...5

Observed Opinion................ . ...

ANNEX 2: Research Protocol Proposal

Research Protocol Proposal

We propose carrying out a double-blind, randomized, controlled study with a quantitative approach, bearing in mind that these are the studies that best allow us to assess the effectiveness of a given therapeutic approach in a population of users. The fact that it is randomized means that the participants selected for the study were chosen at random, i.e. they all have the same probability of belonging to it. The main characteristic of the simple random sample is that it produces samples that are representative of the population and also allows inferential statistics to be used to analyze the data.

Based on these assumptions, two groups of patients will be defined, selected at random and divided into groups A and B. In order for this assumption to be verified, we will draw up a list of all the individuals who come to the clinic with a diagnosis of CFS. The simple random sample consists of drawing up a numerical list of elements from which, with the help of a table of random numbers, a series of numbers are drawn to make up the sample (Fortin, 2009).

We believe that the sample should consist of **100 individuals**.

Group A will be the experimental group where the acupuncture points used for this study will be punctured. The control group will be punctured with sham acupuncture, i.e. the needle will be inserted 1 cun lateral to the real point, diverted from any conduit. In order for the study to be double-blind, neither the subject nor the researcher will be aware of the variables being studied. Thus, acupuncture will be practiced by an acupuncturist external to the study.

As was done in this study, we consider it important that the treatment lasts 4 weeks, with twice-weekly acupuncture sessions.

General objective: To evaluate the effectiveness of acupuncture in controlling the symptoms of CCS.

Inclusion criteria: individuals aged 18 or over; with a medical diagnosis of carpal tunnel syndrome, presence of symptoms lasting more than 3 months, occurring both during the day and at night.

Exclusion criteria: Minors; individuals with another associated pathology, such as rheumatoid arthritis or arthrosis of the hands, or other pathologies that mask the symptoms of the pathology under study.

Study variables:

Dependent variable: Effect of acupuncture on the control of symptoms related to CCS.

Independent Variable: Individuals with CCS undergoing acupuncture treatments.

Instruments used: We consider the Boston self-assessment questionnaire used in this study to be quite adequate and therefore suggest its use.

The Dynamometer should also be used to assess grip strength before and after treatment, as it significantly shows the changes that have occurred as a result of the effect of acupuncture.

We also recommend using a goniometer to assess possible changes in the opening angle of the hand.

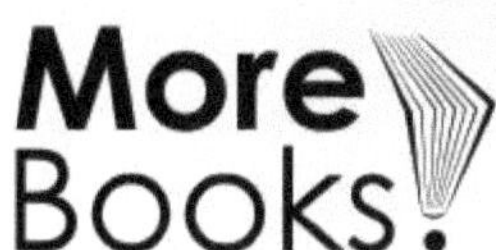

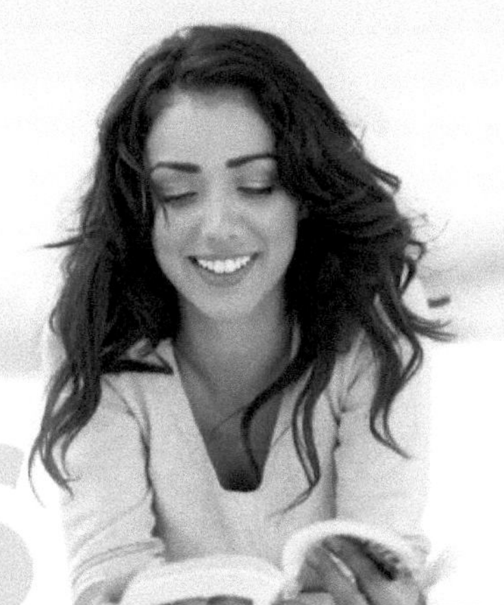

yes
I want morebooks!

Buy your books fast and straightforward online - at one of world's fastest growing online book stores! Environmentally sound due to Print-on-Demand technologies.

Buy your books online at
www.morebooks.shop

Kaufen Sie Ihre Bücher schnell und unkompliziert online – auf einer der am schnellsten wachsenden Buchhandelsplattformen weltweit! Dank Print-On-Demand umwelt- und ressourcenschonend produzi ert.

Bücher schneller online kaufen
www.morebooks.shop

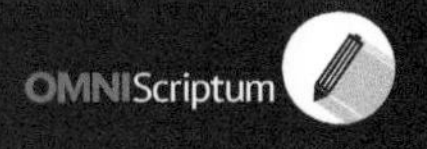

Printed by Books on Demand GmbH, Norderstedt / Germany